OPTIMAL
HEALTH
GUIDELINES
Fourth Edition

by
John R. Lee, M.D.

Sebastopol, CA August 1999

OPTIMAL HEALTH GUIDELINES
Copyright © 1993 by John R. Lee, MD

This book is not intended to replace medical care.
It is intended (1) to be a guide and a knowledge base to help
prevent disease and attain health; (2) to supplement
conventional medical care; and (3) to empower one to become
his/her own best medical advocate. If illness occurs, consult a
physician regarding additional courses of action.

Printed in the United States of America

First printing, August 1993
Second printing, January 1994
Third printing, October 1995 (revised with index)
Fourth printing, October 1999 (revised)

ISBN 0-9643737-0-X

BLL Publishing
P.O. Box 2068
Sebastopol, CA 95473-2068

Cover design © Tu Pham

OPTIMAL HEALTH GUIDELINES

CONTENTS

FORWARD

THIS BOOK, LIKE MANY OTHERS, *derives from a journey. Its subject is health but more than that it concerns a way of looking at what health is. The practice of medicine is a constant learning experience, as any good doctor will tell you. I was not long into the practice of medicine before I realized that my patients were teaching me lessons demanding a different viewpoint than I had learned in medical school. The task of reaching a diagnosis, a name to call their illness, was often quite easy and sometimes quite difficult but always unsatisfying. Too often, a diagnosis is nothing more than a Latin or Greek description of the illness's main symptom (i.e., jaundice = yellowish), sometimes combined with an identification of the main body part involved (i.e., arthritis = inflamed joints); rarely does it speak to cause. I could not help wondering <u>why</u> this particular illness (arthrtitis, pneumonia, cancer, etc.) now afflicts this particular patient. The presence of hemolytic streptococci on a throat culture, for example, does not explain why they succeeded in infecting this particular patient's throat or why they are making her/him so ill. When throat cultures are obtained from people without any apparent illness, the same hemolytic Strep will grow out. Why are these persons carriers of the germ and yet not ill from them? Something more is going on.*

This method of classifying disease by description of some set of signs and symptoms is, of course, long-standing in the history of medicine. However, in the latter half of the past century the discoveries by Louis Pasteur (1822-95) and Robert Koch (1843-1910) of specific microbes as the cause of specific diseases, e.g., anthrax and tuberculosis, an idea initially resisted by their contemporaries, led to the germ theory of disease. With the development of vaccines and, in the present century, the discovery of fungal-derived antibiotics, the single-factor germ theory became a dominating force in medical thinking. The previous mind-set of constitutional, or toxins, or nutritional factors in the etiology of disease states was proportionately demoted and neglected. The "magic bullet" concept of Paul Erlich became the Holy Grail of contemporary medicine and its vision of conquest over disease.

Medicine adopted the metaphor of War: War on the germ invaders; War on Cancer; identify the symptom and find the agent to neutralize it. This seductive paradigm has turned out to be an illusion and an aberration in the history of medicine. Certainly, some of the infectious diseases were successfully treated with vaccines and antibiotics. But this is part of the illusion. More sober analysis finds that simple societal changes such as untainted water and food supplies, proper waste disposal, improved diets, and even the adoption of cotton underwear have probably been the major factors in control of infectious diseases. But even as the antibiotic treated diseases have faded, others have emerged to take their place. Death may not claim the young as it did a century ago, but those of middle age or older are afflicted with a baffling variety of diseases that keep our ever increasing number of doctors busy. The War metaphor no longer applies: our illnesses stem from multiple subtle factors that lead us ever deeper into the workings of our intracellular molecules. We are now in the age of heterogenic molecular disorder and no "magic bullet" will save us. We are forced to return to "constitutional" (i.e., chromososmes) and environmental (e.g., nutritional, avoidance of toxins) factors to understand the plague of viral and degenerative disorders that now predominantly afflict us.

Insight often comes from the little things. In the late 1950s when I opened my office in family practice in Mill Valley, I was visited by an aunt of mine who was seeing California with a female friend, both in their sixties. In the course of our conversation, it was revealed that both had suffered from repeated migraine headaches for many years. Interestingly, one informed me that she had found relief by strictly avoiding citrus fruits and the other prevented her migraines by eating a sliced orange every morning. Another woman, a patient who had suffered "irritable bowel" symptoms for many years, related complete relief when she and her husband had traveled in Mexico where she had discovered the pleasure of eating fresh papaya. She wondered if there was some test to discern whether the clearing of her bowel disorder was the papaya or the freedom from her domestic duties at home. I suggested she could try eating fresh papaya at home. She did and it worked. These and other examples of biochemical individuality abound in medical practice and yet are commonly overlooked. Some years later when I read the books of Roger J. Williams, who describes this phenomenon so well, I could not help but wonder why medical training gives it so little attention.

In most medical schools, various departments are identified by a specific body organ, e.g., cardiology, nephrology, dermatology, orthopedics (bones and joints), neurology, gastroenterology, etc. The student is presented with a medical paradigm that catalogues disease states by the organ most prominently afflicted. More recent advances will move the cataloging practice to some smaller portion of an organ, e.g., coronary arteries, bronchitis versus pneumonitis, tendonitis versus bursitis, etc. Until rather recently, cancers were identified by the organ from which they arose, e.g., bone cancer, liver cancer, etc.; only since the mid 1970s has there been an attempt to identify cancer by cell type rather than organ site. It should be apparent now that disease is a manifestation of molecular disorder in the complex workings at the intracellular level, a malfunctioning of the marvelous balancing act going on deep within the billions of cells of which our body is made. The old unifactorial paradigm no longer pertains.

The new paradigm of understanding health and disease was described in the 1973 book, "Predictive Medicine: A Study in Strategy," by Drs. E. Cheraskin and WM. Ringsdorf, Jr., in which the superficial signs and symptoms of a disease were seen only as outward manifestations of a deeper underlying intracellular disorder. The disease, as it presents itself, is the result of physiologic problems brought on by biochemical imbalance, hormonal imbalance, and/or enzyme imbalance due to a multi-factorial variety of destabilizing factors (nutritional, toxic, traumatic. etc.) being dealt with to varying degrees of success by genetically determined physico-chemical characteristics of the living organism. Cheraskin's and Ringsdorf's book was, and continues to be, a vision of how medical concepts should be viewed.

From this new paradigm flow concepts of gradation (i.e., degree of disease rather than a presumed presence or absence of disease), homeostasis (the body's ability to maintain a stable internal environment), biochemical individuality, and a spectrum of interactions and possible outcomes rather than the earlier presumed simple linear relationships. The same "disease" in two people may stem from entirely different causes (cardiomyopathy from a virus, magnesium deficiency, or alcohol abuse). Similarly, the same "cause" may result in different "diseases" in two different people (e.g. zinc deficiency may appear only as white spots in fingernails in one person, delayed wound healing in another, or enteropathy in still another). The organ system specialist may recognize a nutritional deficiency effect in the organ function of his specialty but will likely not recognize the same deficiency as it presents itself in other organ systems. In treating osteoporosis, for example, the orthopedist is inclined to assign his patients a different therapy than would a gynecologist or an internist. Each of them approaches the problem from his specialty's perspective. It is time for the new paradigm that approaches health from an orthomolecular viewpoint.

The old unifactorial paradigm is still found in contemporary medicine. Doctors will argue whether ulcers, for example, are caused by stress, diet, hyper-acidity, or by the recently accepted acid-loving bacterium, Helicobacter pylori. They do not readily opt for the possibility that all of these factors interact to cause the problem. Similarly, doctors debate whether a particular disease is "functional" or "organic," not realizing that the distinction is illusory. They have been taught to seek out the cause rather than seek to understand the multiple interrelationships at work. Even with infections, once so easily treated with antibiotics, we see that the old paradigm fails. With the advent of AIDS it has become obvious to all that the immune competency of the host is a major determinant of the disease's course. In fact, it is now abundantly evident that no amount of antibiotic therapy can cure an immune-deficient patient of TB; one's "constitution" is indeed important.

Unifactorial thinking is especially pervasive in medical research where the "double blind" test has become the gold standard. When each individual is recognized to be biochemically and physiologically different from every other person and, in addition, when each disease is seen as a result of multiple factors operating within a complex interreacting system, the strategy for dealing with matters of health becomes undesirably muddied for linear thinkers. This, however, is reality. To think and act otherwise is to become a character in a Lewis Carrol Alice in Wonderland fantasy wherein the Red Queen can alter reality at will. Fortunately, the multiple factors relating to the prevention of one disease are found to be the same among the majority of other diseases, i.e., health in all senses has common factors which pertain to the large majority of diseases at which we are at risk. Understanding these factors is the focus of this book.

Finally, it must be recognized that medicine is an immature science with great areas presently unknown. We are on a learning curve and this presents a problem. At what point along this curve should one be so audacious as to present his picture of the knowledge he has acquired? It is similar, one might suppose, to a navigator making a chart or drawing a map. He has completed a journey and made some discoveries along a route he has come. He wishes to show others the shoals to avoid and the path of clear sailing so he draws his map despite the areas still unknown. Perhaps future explorers will find a better route, will navigate other areas of the sea, will mark the currents and shoals along even more distant ports of call; but the map he charts will be an improvement on what existed before. That is reason enough for the map he draws. So it is with this book. The accumulating body of knowledge now leads us to a different paradigm, a new understanding of health, and hopefully better routes of travel in our passage through life. Use this book as you would the chart of the navigator who wishes you clear sailing.

John R. Lee, MD

INTRODUCTION

OPTIMAL HEALTH MEANS BEING IN the best possible health one can be within the constraints of genetic and constitutional limitations. One's health is a product of a many factors of which nutrition, exercise, and techniques for dealing with stress are the major factors under one's own control. This book is an outline of the present available knowledge, the understanding of which can serve as a guideline to anyone interested in his or her optimal health goals.

The lessons and explanations of health matters embodied herein have been derived from over four decades of study and medical practice emphasizing the preventive aspects of health care. Contemporary medicine in the US is the world leader in the treatment of acute illness, trauma, and surgery. However, it is only recently that attention is being directed to preventive health concepts, especially those that apply to support of molecular health. The typical physician's education and standard practice precepts follow a pattern of diagnosis by physical signs and patient symptoms, augmented by an array of laboratory and radiological tests, which then lead to more or less standardized treatment programs directed at the diagnosis reached. Only rarely are the underlying physiological malfunctions that precede the diagnostic signs and symptoms sought or even considered. The result is a "cookbook" approach to medical care which, though much admired by middle managers of health care systems, leads to stagnation in health research and the ultimate failure of disease prevention. Those physicians seeking to understand and correct the deeper underlying causes of disease by finding ways to restore healthy cellular function or proper molecular balance tend to find themselves labeled as "alternative" physicians, an appellation somehow weighted by medical orthodoxy with negative connotations.

When one reviews the results of treatment by contemporary medicine, one is struck by several interesting findings. One is that the vast majority of illnesses treated, such as arthritis, hypertension, coronary heart disease, etc., are not cured, per se, but merely kept under some degree of control by our treatments, with progression or recurrence of the illness a likely matter. The other is that, of the illnesses that are truly cured, such as pernicious anemia, scurvy, rickets, beriberi, iron deficiency anemia, pellagra, etc., one finds they are all caused by a simple deficiency of one or another vital nutrient. It should not be beyond imagination that many more, if not most, illnesses result in large part from nutritional factors.

Furthermore, the typical patient (and his/her physician) is often unaware that most of our successful medical treatments have their origin in natural compounds and sold to us as "drugs." Antibiotics, antimalarials, antiarthritis pills, antihypertensives, anti-cancer drugs, anti-gout medications, analgesics, anti-oxidants and many others have come to us from natural sources. It is probable that we have only begun to discover the magic of Nature's medicine box.

Stress, whether physical, physiological or psychological, can be helpful or harmful depending on its force and our adaptation to it. There are lessons to be learned in coping with stress. Helmets for cyclists, drivers training, seat belts, or training for safe scuba diving seem obvious preventive health measures; but a similar training for coping with psychological stresses is rarely addressed except in retrospect. Understanding the physiologic mechanisms and the wide range of potential consequences of stress, and learning adequate coping techniques, are just as important as automobile seat belts and driver training classes.

Exercise in the course of daily activities has been, until the present century, the standard condition of human existence. With the advent of the automobile, washing machines and other "labor-saving" machines, many of us lead a life with little exercise. This decline in exercise has broad physiologic consequences, most of which are negative. Under-exercised and undeveloped muscles will fail us earlier as we age. Coronary artery capacity remains smaller and thus more likely to occlude in those persons growing up with less exercise. Connective tissue and even our bones are stronger if we exercise. Poor musculature leads to poor lung power with consequent loss of tissue oxygenation and more rapid aging. The list of the many problems stemming from poor exercise is long, as might be imagined. The good news is that proper exercise, at any age, brings positive benefits.

A healthy life is one's most treasured gift but it requires some tending to. It rarely comes to someone who ignores the lessons of Nature, especially in the circumstances of our present environment. Good health requires proper choices in the matter of what we eat and how we live. It is the goal of this book to provide a knowledge base for the making of these choices.

This book is a guideline, not an encyclopedia, for health. But once the basic concepts and fundamentals are understood, and the application of them undertaken, the benefits will follow. Later, as further knowledge unfolds, additional refinements can be easily adapted. The care and tending of optimal health is a continual life process, a path of enlightenment, empowerment and joy which returns the responsibility for health to the proper party, you. Each one of us carves but a single path through life. Why not make it a healthy one?

PREFACE

THIS BOOK WAS ORIGINALLY WRITTEN as a course book for a class entitled Optimal Health that I teach at College of Marin, The sixteen chapters match the sixteen weekly class meetings through two terms each year. The demand for the books, however, exceeded the size of the class and numerous requests have been received for extra copies. To accommodate readers outside of my class, I have added an introduction and a forward to provide information normally presented during class and have re-formatted the pages and type for easier reading.

The book is divided into two sections, corresponding to the two eight-week school terms during which the class meets. The first section, Optimal Health Concepts and Fundamentals, deals with nutrition, stress, and exercise, the three factors which seem to me to be the most important health factors more or less under our own control. The second section, Optimal Health Applications, applies these lessons to a number of our major health concerns. Following the second section is a glossary of unavoidable medical terms that should be useful for the non-medical reader who may not be familiar with them. The purpose of the book is to serve as a guideline to good health, empowering each reader with knowledge by which he can regain responsibility for his/her own optimal health decisions and choices.

The little quizzes at the end of each chapter are meant to provide a means of checking on your own reading of each chapter and, hopefully, to be a bit amusing. The answers can be found at the end of each of the two major book sections.

Good reading and optimal health to you all!

OPTIMAL HEALTH:

CONCEPTS & FUNDAMENTALS

Description: An investigation and exposition of basic health concepts and the fundamentals of nutrition, stress, and exercise.

Chapter 1. Introduction to the basic concepts of health; a conceptual model will be developed to understand the relationship of factors destructive to good health and those that defend and restore health.

Chapter 2. This chapter will cover fundamentals of carbohydrates: how these apply to the foods we eat and their effects on health. Learn the important difference between simple and complex carbohydrates.

Chapter 3. Fundamentals of dietary fat and its metabolism. Learn the truth about cholesterol, "cis-" versus "trans-" fatty acids, the problems of processed fats, and the danger of oxidized fat.

Chapter 4. Nutrition study will continue with fundamentals of amino acids and protein metabolism, the importance of proper daily protein intake, and the errors of the standard American diet.

Chapter 5. Nutrition study will conclude with discussion of vitamins, minerals, other micronutrients and fiber. Particular emphasis will be directed to the importance of potassium/sodium balance and its role in hypertension.

Chapter 6. Part One: The Limbic Brain - how our body controls and maintains healthy metabolism and normal body function.

Part Two: The Stress of Life - what stress is and what can we do about it.

Chapter 7. Fundamentals of exercise and the important role it plays in multiple aspects of optimal health.

Chapter 8. The lessons of chapters 1-7 will be reviewed to demonstrate their inter-connectedness in relation to common illnesses in our society. Guidelines to proper diet and optimal health will emerge.

CHAPTER ONE
WHAT IS HEALTH?

Health is not merely the absence of disease. Health is the sum total of our well being at any given moment in our life. Nature provides us with a magnificent set of physiological processes by which we can grow and sustain our bodies in an optimal manner even within the rather wide ranges of circumstances man may choose to live his life. Nature's intent is not to serve only the needs of man, however, but contains many elements, which threaten his health. A simple formula expresses this relationship.

$$\text{HEALTH} = \frac{\text{Processes favorable to man}}{\text{Processes deleterious to man}}$$

What do we mean by processes deleterious to man? These would include infectious agents, toxic compounds, trauma, malnutrition, excessive fatigue, excessive stress, lack of exercise, certain electromagnetic radiations, genetic errors, and even age.

Processes favorable to man would include protection against infection, our success in avoiding toxic agents and/or detoxifying them, learning to avoid unnecessary trauma, securing proper nutrition, rest and exercise, coping with stress, and learning skills and preventive therapies to compensate for genetic error.

Health, then, is optimized by maximizing the favorable processes and minimizing the deleterious ones.

UNDERSTANDING BIOLOGICAL PROCESSES
1. "Linear" vs "Global" thinking
   a. Linear thinking is represented by A $\rightarrow$ B $\rightarrow$ C $\rightarrow$ D. As example, cold germs can cause runny noses, congestion and cough. Common

"treatments" are decongestants and cough suppressants, which disguise symptoms but ignore the cause, which is an inadequate immune response to the cold virus. Another example is heart disease that can cause a watery swelling (edema) of the ankles. Linear thinking results in treatment (taking a drug) that increases one's kidney excretion of water but does nothing for one's heart. A third example might be hypertension in which the pressure of blood being pumped through our arteries is too high. With linear thinking, treatment might be drugs that (a) weaken our heart action {beta blockers}, or (b) dilate our arteries {calcium channel blockers or vasodilators} or (c) decrease the watery portion of our blood volume by tricking the kidneys into excreting more water {diuretics}.

As you can see, linear thinking treats symptoms, i.e., the superficial manifestations of the disease, as if they were the disease itself. It does not get to the heart of the problem.

b. Global thinking is the attempt to see and work with the true nature of the problem. In the case of colds, we know that cold germs are always around us. We "catch" colds when our resistance is down, the viruses attack cell membranes of our respiratory system, i.e., nose, sinuses, and bronchial tree. We can increase our resistance to cold germs by maintaining proper vitamins C and A, by proper rest and exercise, and by adequate hydration (water intake). We can use niacin (vitamin B3) to liquefy nasal or sinus mucus rather than antihistamines that will thicken mucus and cause drowsiness; and we can understand that catching a few colds early in life builds up our immune defenses. In the case of fluid retention in heart disease, we can learn about the dynamics of sodium and potassium loads and discover that fluid accumulation occurs whenever the proper ratio of sodium to potassium is exceeded. The same is true in most cases of hypertension. Optimal health requires learning the knack of global thinking.

2. A deeper look at global thinking

a. The nature of physiologic processes is not unlike what we see occurring globally on Earth. Floods, drought, pestilence, and earthquakes are merely local superficial reflections of what is occurring at some deeper level of Earth processes. So it is in matters of health.

Let us look at a typical living cell of which our bodies have 60 trillion or so. Each has an enclosing membrane and inside is a nucleus with 46 chromosomes from which messenger RNA bring the orders of function to minute organs within the cell's interior (cytoplasm). Intracellular organelles (the mitochondria) build energy molecules from glucose; hormones are synthesized; and enzymes (>2000 different types per cell), some of which build specific molecules needed by the body and others dismember foreign or toxic molecules. The cell sits in a watery milieu from which its cell membrane selectively absorbs nutrients or restricts intake of toxins; and excretes waste products of its own metabolism. The cell cytoplasm and its enveloping membrane have entry sites ("receptor sites") for messages carried by circulating hormones; and chemical "pumps" for maintaining the proper balance of minerals and salts for the necessary catalysts and building material. Some cells (e.g., white blood cells) are motile and actively seek out invaders to destroy. Some cells exist only to reproduce other cells that wear out and need to be replaced (e.g., red blood cells, skin cells, etc.). Others (e.g., nerve and muscle cells) never reduplicate themselves and, when they suffer enough damage to be killed, are lost forever. Each is immensely intricate and is a complex miracle of life.

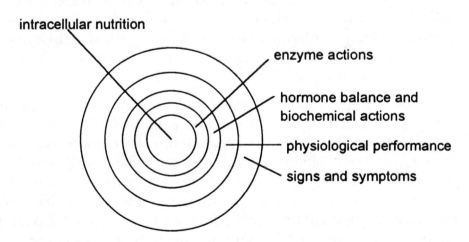

intracellular nutrition

enzyme actions

hormone balance and biochemical actions

physiological performance

signs and symptoms

Global view of the importance of nutrition to health.

(7)

Global thinking requires that we look at the metabolic processes as they extend from the intracellular organs to cell function to organ function to physiologic function and eventually to health itself. And beyond all that, we must think in terms of the nutrients needed by the cell and of the agents to which we are exposed that can interfere with cell activity.

b. The example of vitamin A. All yellow and dark green vegetables contain betacarotene, which we absorb and circulate through our bodies. Each of our cells can convert betacarotene to vitamin A using an enzyme which itself is dependent on zinc as a catalyst. If zinc is deficient, our production of vitamin A will be deficient. Vitamin A is necessary for our vision's adaptation to darkness, cell membrane integrity (especially of the mucous lining cells of our respiratory system and intestinal system), strong skin, the protective exterior lining (conjunctiva) of our eyes, and normal reproduction. Therefore, zinc deficiency might show itself as various forms of vitamin A deficiency such as night blindness or any of the following: acne, eczema, eye infections, colds and other respiratory infections, emphysema or bronchiectasis or lung cancer (in smokers), diarrhea, colon cancer, and other cancers. In North Africa, blindness from fly-carried chlamydial eye infections was virtually eliminated by adding yellow vegetables or vitamin A to the children's diets. In South Africa, child deaths due to measles pneumonia were reduced by over 50% by timely supplementation of vitamin A, irrespective of their initial serum vitamin A levels. Treating the superficial symptoms does not work; treating the cause is the key.

In the example above, the linear thinker might conclude that all patients low in zinc or vitamin A should acquire all of the above. The global thinker will understand that numerous other processes are also at work, some increasing the risks of some particular damage and some working with the body to prevent damage. Each of us is an individual with differing sets of life factors including genetic, nutritional, toxic exposures, emotional stress, other illnesses, etc., etc. No element operates strictly alone; each is a component of a matrix, some enhancing the effect of another element (synergy) and some impairing another's function (antagonist). Consider the example of music. It is composed of individual notes but the beauty and the effect emanates from how they blend together. It is no different in the orchestration of the body's functioning.

WHICH KIND OF MEDICAL CARE DO YOU WANT?
FINDING THE ANSWER

1. The way of conventional medicine

Think of your body as your home; disease agents sneak into your body through cracks in your defenses, like rats or termites sneaking into your home. Conventional medicine supplies you with traps and poisons to kill the vermin or termites. Conventional medicine follows the metaphor of war: the disease agent is an enemy to be killed. As in your home, poisons that kill vermin or termites can also be a threat to you. And killing one rat does not prevent others from sneaking through the same cracks.

2. The way of Optimal Health

Optimal health follows the way, not of war, but of healing; healing the cracks in your home, your body. Defense against disease and the healing powers of your body are greater than any drug. Keep your house in order and the rats and termites can not invade. All your body requires is the proper mix of nutrition, exercise, and mental attitude. That is the way of optimal health.

At first glance, the prospect of ever understanding global thinking and arriving at appropriate decisions in our search for optimal health may seem overwhelmingly complicated and unreachable. But here Mother Nature has made our course considerably easier than might be expected. It turns out that broad general principles underlie and are applicable to a great variety of illnesses (especially the so-called "degenerative" diseases) and that our understanding of these general principles can lead to a simplified approach beneficial to all of them. Elucidating these general principles will be the main emphasis of this course. This, in turn, will lead to a pattern of decision-making in life's choices that can optimize health at any age or stage of health.

CHAPTER ONE

When you go to your doctor, keep in mind the following question. Does your doctor look into possible causes, or does he/she merely add up your symptoms and then reach for the prescription pad? Ask your doctor about your prescriptions. Are they meant to treat the cause of your illness, or are they meant only to relieve some of the symptoms. Remember, the symptoms are not the disease: they are the outward manifestation of the disease. It is up to you to get your doctor to think of finding and treating causes, not the symptoms. If he/she is reluctant or will not take the time to do that, find a better doctor.

It is important to first recognize that we constantly make choices in life: choices of diet, of activities, of dealing with stress, even what music we listen to and what clothes we wear. Then we must recognize that there are consequences of the choices we make. When we acquire knowledge of these consequences, we then have the advantage of being able to make the right choices for obtaining optimal health. The decision of doing so or not is then up to each individual.

Note: Well-researched studies indicate that in the US, *preventable illness makes up approximately 70 % of the burden of disease and the associated costs.* When causes of death are classified by underlying actual causes rather than traditional disease-oriented diagnoses, it is found that *preventable causes account for eight of the nine leading categories and for 980,000 deaths per year.* What could be more clear?

*from *NEJM*, 29 July 1993, vol. 329, no. 5, pgs 321-325.

SELF-QUIZ

This is an opportunity to review what was discussed in chapter 1.

1. Antihistamines are good treatments for viral upper respiratory infections. True or False?

2. If you take a good vitamin supplement, you can eat anything you want. True or False?

3. Heart disease is largely hereditary and there isn't much you can do about it. True or False?

4. We build up our immune defenses by avoiding germs as much as possible. True or False?

5. If you are feeling generally pretty good, it means your diet is fine. True or False?

6. Most of us are as healthy as can be expected. True or False?

7. When you get sick, the doctor's medicines will generally make you well. True or False?

8. If you keep catching colds, it's not your fault. True or False?

9. Eating correctly is boring and too much trouble. True or False?

10. When we get older, we have to expect to be less healthy. True of False?

Answers to questions are on page 85.

CHAPTER TWO
CARBOHYDRATES

Nutrition refers to the nourishment of living organisms for growth, energy and repair. Our bodies need air (oxygen), water, and food. Scientists look at food and see carbohydrates, fats, and proteins plus certain minerals, vitamins, and other micronutrients. The rest of us look at food and see only vegetables, fruit, meat, dairy products, nuts, baked goods, eggs, and fish and other seafood. Scientists tell us to eat certain fatty acids and to avoid others, to limit fat intake to less than 30% of our calories, to eat a "balanced" diet, and to limit sodium to less than 3 gm/day; but somehow that doesn't tell us what to put on our grocery list. The question we face is: what should we know about carbohydrates and how do we go about doing it right? The answer to this question is the theme of chapter 2.

CARBOHYDRATES

Carbohydrates are relatively simple molecules composed of carbon, hydrogen, and oxygen. They are synthesized by plants from carbon dioxide (from the air) and water, utilizing energy they derive from sunlight, a process we call photosynthesis. The simplest are sugars (monosaccharides) which are composed of 6 carbon atoms, 12 hydrogen atoms, and 6 oxygen atoms, i.e., 6 carbons and 6 water molecules. Some sugars (e.g. sucrose, maltose, lactose) are made of two simple sugars put together. They are called disaccharides. One disaccharide (lactose) is made in mammals' breasts by combining two simple sugars, and is found in milk: it is the only sugar available from an animal source.

Plants can link many simple sugars together in long chains (polymers) we call starch, as in grain starch or potatoes, or, when finely ground, we refer to them as flour. When we eat them, they don't taste like sugar because our salivary enzyme (ptyalin, a.k.a., salivary amylase) does not cleave them into separate sugars; but, in the stomach, they quickly dissolve into simple sugars which we then absorb.

Some plants combine the sugar molecules into more complex cross-linked polymer formations for rigidity and strength; these we call cellulose. The simpler forms of these, found in vegetables and fruit (e.g. apples), are digestible by humans. More highly cross-linked forms, such as the cellulose in grass and grain stalks, are digestible only by grazing animals. Wood cellulose is indigestible to all except a unique and complex protozoan-like organism, *Myxotricha paradoxa*, that lives in the stomach of termites.

Examples of the molecular formation of two simple sugars and a disaccharide are pictured below.

Glucose

Fructose
(crystallized)

Galactose   Glucose

Lactose

When broken down (hydrolyzed) to simple sugars, carbohydrates are absorbed without further digestion. Sugar is the primary fuel for the energy needed by most cells. Sugars not used quickly for energy demands are stored for future use, usually by being converted into fat, which is a much more efficient form of energy storage. (13 lbs of sugar can be converted into 1 lb of fat for storage. That allows us to carry around a good supply of energy without being as heavy as a tree.) A small amount of sugar (3 oz or so) is stored in the liver as glycogen, a polysaccharide which, when needed for energy, can be returned to the blood as glucose. We do not have an efficient way of excreting excess sugar: the kidney will do its best to excrete excess sugar in the urine but that mechanism operates only when blood sugar exceeds a higher threshold level, e.g., as in diabetes. In general, eating more sugar or starch than needed for energy will make you fat.

When sugar is metabolized for energy, the waste products are carbon dioxide (CO_2) and water. We breath out the carbon dioxide (so plants can use it again) and excrete the water in urine. It is a clean burning fuel, which, if not used as such within a few minutes (15-30) after eating, will be converted into fat for storage. The more complex starches require more digestion time to be converted into sugars so, therefore, their ability to nourish the body extends over a longer period of time than the simple sugars.

The bacteria (*Strep mutans*) that live in dental plaque metabolize sugar and starch in our food. They convert it into an acid that dissolves the dental enamel, thus causing cavities (dental caries). Lactose in milk is especially prone to this action.

Sugars taste sweet and are found mostly in fruits. Starches are taste-less and are found in grains (wheat, rice, corn, etc.), tubers (e.g., pota-toes), and, in smaller amounts, in many other vegetables. Some plant sugars are put together in fibers that we can not digest. They are impor-tant in their own way and will be discussed separately. (See chapter 5.)

DIGESTION AND ABSORPTION OF CARBOHYDRATES

The digestion of sugar and starch starts in the mouth with an enzyme (ptyalin, or salivary amylase) found in saliva. Salivary amy-lase is inactivated by stomach acid. The simple sugars, like alcohol, are absorbed into the blood without requiring any gastric digestion. Fructose is more slowly absorbed than other monosaccharides such as glucose and galactose. Starch and the disaccharides such as su-crose, lactose and maltose that were not hydrolyzed and absorbed in the stomach then pass through to the duodenum where their hy-drolysis is completed by pancreatic amylase, leading to their prompt absorption. Complex carbohydrates such as grains and vegetable cellulose require the longest time for eventual absorption. Glucose is the primary fuel for cellular energy, providing 4 Kcal of energy per gram (fats provide 9 Kcal per gram).

The sweet taste of sugar stimulates the beta cells of the pancreas to secrete the important enzyme, insulin, which facilitates this cellular process of sugar metabolism (except for fructose). Though sugars are the simplest of foods, the energy-releasing process involves a number of other enzymes, each of which requires specific mineral and vitamin co-factors (catalysts). Since sugar provides none of these other essential factors, it is commonly referred to as "empty calories." Also, whenever cellular intake of sugar exceeds metabolic need, sugar is converted into fat for storage.

The disaccharides found in the typical diet are sucrose, lactose (from milk) and maltose. They are composed of glucose + fructose, glucose + galactose, and glucose + glucose, respectively. The enzyme for digesting the milk sugar, lactose, is ß-galactosidase (also called lactase) and is normally present in humans only during infancy and childhood, allowing the young to acquire energy from the sugar in mothers' milk. Because of genetic predisposition or adaptation, this enzyme persists in northern European children until middle age, allowing the use of cows' milk by adults. Most of the world's population lives in the equatorial zone where plant foods are available the year around and cows' milk is neither available nor necessary. In northern climes, such foods did not exist in winter; sustenance in winter depended on cow or goat milk.

Milk consumed at an age when lactase is not present for digestion is thus not absorbed and not available for energy. The lactose passes undigested through the stomach and intestines to the colon where colon bacteria ferment it with their own enzymes, usually causing rectal gas and feelings of indigestion. Young blacks and Asians, even after several generations in the US, still lose their lactase in mid-teens and experience this form of indigestion when drinking milk or eating ice cream. The technique of adding a live culture into milk for a benign fermentation of the lactose allows adults to drink milk without this risk of lactose intolerance. Such products are yogurt, kefir, and buttermilk.

Artificial sweeteners are not saccharides but are chemical compounds that stimulate a sweet taste as sugar does. If one uses artificial sweeteners, the tongue detects the sweet taste of sugar and the same secretion of insulin ensues with the result that normally present blood sugar is transferred into fat and muscle cells. If not used for energy, this sugar is converted into fat, as mentioned above. The falling blood sugar level creates a sense of hunger and a desire to eat more. In test animals, such artificial sweeteners added to the diet will cause obesity, lassitude, and a general inability to cope. It is perversely ironic that they are advertised as a putative benefit for diabetics and for obesity. These artificial sweeteners now constitute about 20% of the "sugar" sales in the US.

In addition, the sugar substitute, aspartame, is unique in that it consists of a compound of two amino acids, phenylalanine and aspartic acid , combined as a methyl ester. When stored in liquid, e.g., canned drinks, some of the aspartame converts to methyl alcohol, which is neuro- and nephro-toxic. When aspartame is metabolized in body cells, the concentration of these two amino acids can reach abnormally high levels. This is especially disconcerting in the central nervous system where these amino acids can influence the synthesis of various neuro-transmitters leading to neurological abnormalities. The problems associated with aspartame (trade name NutraSweet) have been catalogued by HJ Roberts, MD, and include headaches, eye problems, psychiatric problems, epileptic seizures, brain tumors, and Alzheimer's disease. Further, Dr. Roberts' review of the history of aspartame's approval by the Food and Drug Administration (FDA) finds that it was suspiciously lax and suggests an overriding industrial influence. As should be obvious, artificial sweeteners are not conducive to good health. (See chapter 13, the discussion of Alzheimer's disease.)

PHYSIOLOGIC ASPECTS OF CARBOHYDRATE METABOLISM

After digestion and absorption, carbohydrates are carried in the bloodstream as glucose and/or fructose. The concentration of glucose is normally regulated by the body to remain within the range of 70-110 mg/dl. This regulation involves the interaction of several complex functions primarily under the control of the liver, pancreas, kidney, and endocrine glands (thyroid, pituitary, adrenal). The pancreas secretes two hormones, insulin and glucagon, that are important in this regulation process. A rise in glucose concentration triggers the release of insulin that facilitates absorption of blood glucose into

(17)

body cells for cellular energy. Insulin also increases the conversion of glucose not used for energy into fat. In this manner, insulin prevents blood glucose concentrations from rising above the desired range. Fructose is different in that its absorption and utilization is independent of insulin.

Glucagon, made by the pancreas in the case of low blood glucose concentrations, raises blood glucose levels. It stimulates the release of glucose (stored in the liver as glycogen) and promotes the synthesis of glucose from protein (a process called gluconeogenesis). Glucagon also enables the body to use stored fat for energy instead of glucose. Thus, glucagon prevents blood glucose levels from falling below the desired range.

Blood glucose concentrations below the normal range (hypoglycemia) stimulate the release of adrenaline, which is a quick-acting method for releasing liver glycogen into the blood as glucose. In some people, especially as a result of prolonged stress, insulin release is greater than needed and leads to reactive hypoglycemia. That is, a rapid rise of blood glucose (by eating sugar and refined starch) is followed by a rather rapid fall in blood glucose levels that trigger an adrenalin response to restore glucose levels. This will be discussed more thoroughly in following chapters.

Elevated cortisol (as in stress or Cushing's disease) also will elevate blood glucose levels. Excess thyroid hormone, on the other hand, increases the metabolic rate, thereby increasing the body's rate of metabolizing glucose for energy.

Certain medications disrupt the normal regulation of blood glucose. Low blood glucose can result from anti-diabetes drugs (e.g., tolbutamide, tolazamide, acetohexamide, chlorpropramide, glyburide, or glipizide) and also from pentamidine (frequently used to treat pneumonia in AIDS patients).

Hypoglycemia that occurs in a person who has not eaten for 12 hours or so suggests the possibility of abnormally low functioning of the thyroid, pituitary, or adrenal gland, or, more rarely, the presence of a pancreatic insulin-producing tumor.

As described above, simple carbohydrates such as sugar and refined starch are unique among foods in being absorbed quickly into the blood stream creating a surge of blood sugar. Such simple carbohydrates are found only in relatively small amounts in unprocessed foods. The sugar content of a can of Coca-Cola or Pepsi Cola, for example, is about 9 teaspoons of crystallized sugar. To ingest an equivalent amount of sugar by eating sugar cane would require over 30 feet of sugar cane! At the turn of the century, the average consumption of sugar in the US was approximately 2 lbs per year; the average consumption of sugar 60 years later rose to over 100 lbs per year. Many teenagers ingest 300 lbs per year, almost one pound per day.

As one might imagine, the human body has difficulty adapting to such a large intake of sugar. This poses a risk not only to persons with diabetes or obesity problems but also to the great majority of those who are presumed to be in good health. Man's ability to metabolize sugar derived from evolutionary times when such sugars were ingested only in much smaller amounts. The present intake of sugar exceeds our innate physiologic capacity and, as such, is toxic. Recent dietary guidelines recommend that sugar should not exceed 5% of daily caloric intake. This will be discussed more thoroughly in chapters 6 and 13.

Complex carbohydrates (grains, seeds, and vegetables) do not share this potential hazard since they require prolonged digestion and absorption, and thus do not lead to the blood sugar surge found after ingesting the simple sugars. Complex carbohydrates provide our major source of energy and should make up a major portion of our daily caloric intake.

THE GLYCEMIC INDEX

After digestion and absorption from the intestine, glucose circulates in blood. A rising blood glucose level stimulates insulin production. As indicated above, insulin lowers blood glucose concentration by increasing glucose transport into the tissue cells, particularly those of muscle and adipose (fat) tissue. It also promotes the storage of glucose in these tissues either as glycogen (muscle) or as triacylglycerols (triglyceride) in fat. The greater the surge of glucose into blood, the greater is the production of insulin. As described above, some carbohydrates require more digestion time than others do. Simple sugars are absorbed faster than complex carbohydrates. Thus, simple sugars produce a greater surge of glucose into blood and a greater production of insulin. Food items can be ranked by their insulin response. This is called the glycemic index. Those foods that cause higher production of insulin are said to have a higher glycemic index. In this ranking, glucose is given a glycemic index of 100. Foods that cause a greater insulin response will have a glycemic index higher than 100, and those foods that cause less of an insulin response are ranked lower than 100.

For example, puffed rice and rice cakes are ranked the highest, at a glycemic index of 133. Oatmeal is ranked at 78, and plums have a ranking of 25. Processing of food makes a difference, also. The glycemic index of vegetables generally rises when they are cooked. This is probably related to the heat-induced breakdown of fiber or the cellulose content of the food, releasing the sugar of the food for faster absorption. Flour is more glycemic than the grain from which it was derived. "Instant" oatmeal or instant rice are more glycemic than regular oatmeal or rice. The glycemic effect of sugars and refined carbohydrates (cookies, cake, and other pastries) is greater when they are eaten by themselves than when eaten with fats and proteins. Fructose is the exception to the high glycemic index of sugars. It is a sugar that does not require insulin for absorption into body cells and its glycemic index is only 26.

The difference in glycemic index is very important to health. Many diabetics tolerate food with a low glycemic index ranking such as complex carbohydrates rather than sugar or refined starches. Highly glycemic food is more likely to cause obesity than food with a low glycemic index ranking. Highly glycemic foods are more potent in causing elevated cholesterol levels than are fats. They are more likely to stimulate reactive hypoglycemia. Highly glycemic foods may lead to insulin resistance and thus may cause Type 2 (so-called non-insulin dependent) diabetes. Insulin stimulates growth of cancer cells. In fact, there are a host of symptoms and illnesses (Syndrome X) that result from high surges of insulin and insulin resistance.

The message of all this is simple. Sugar and highly refined carbohydrates are not well tolerated by the body. One is well advised to avoid them and eat carbohydrates the way Mother Nature made them – whole and unrefined.

Remember: All absorbed carbohydrates are eventually metabolized as glucose. When metabolized for energy, the ultimate waste products are CO_2 and H_2O. Only a relatively small amount of glucose is stored in the liver as glycogen. All glucose not metabolized for energy or stored as glycogen is usually converted to FAT. Thus, ingested sugar not needed for energy $\rightarrow$ fat.

SELF QUIZ

1. Sugar is the basic fuel for cellular energy. True or False?

2. Sugar is correctly known as "empty calories." True or False?

3. Starch is made of sugar molecules. True or False?

4. Ingested sugar in excess of need is stored as fat. True or False?

5. Cellulose is made of sugar molecules. True or False?

6. Ounce for ounce, sugar provides less than half as much energy as fat. True or False?

7. Artificial sweeteners can be harmful. True or False?

8. Insulin levels increase just by tasting sugar. True or False?

9. Complex carbohydrates are all eventually absorbed as sugar. True or False?

10. Complex carbohydrates are better for you than plain sugar. True or False?

Answers can be found on page 85.

CHAPTER THREE

FATS AND OILS (LIPIDS)

Fats and oils are, like carbohydrates, also made of carbon, hydrogen and oxygen but their form is a bit different. They are put together in linear linkages, like chains, whereas sugars are constructed more in rings. The carbon atoms are linked to one another and attached to each are the hydrogen atoms. At the end of the chain of carbon atoms, the last carbon is linked to two oxygens and one hydrogen (actually a double-bonded oxygen and a hydroxyl radical made of one oxygen and one hydrogen) which, in organic chemistry, is why it is called a *fatty acid*. In any case, fat contains less oxygen for any given number of carbons than sugars do. That is why they pack together so well for storage. Most stored fat consists of three fatty acids linked to a glycerin molecule and, in that form, they are collectively called triacylglycerols (commonly known as triglycerides).

Saturated fatty acid

Triglyceride

By convention, we refer to lipids that are solid at room temperature as "fat" and, those that are liquid at room temperature, we call "oil." Both are fats. Fats in which all the available carbon valence sites are filled with hydrogen are called *saturated* and tend to be solids. Fatty acids that have double bonds between adjacent carbon atoms (and two less hydrogen atoms) are called *unsaturated*. If only one pair of carbons is double bonded, it is called *monounsaturated*, and those with more than one are called *polyunsaturated*. These fats are more slippery and appear as oils. Also, short chain fatty acids are more likely to be oil and longer chains tend to be solid fat.

Polyunsaturated fatty acid

The location in the molecule of the double-bonded carbons makes a slight bend in the molecule, altering the shape of the fatty acid. This affects the combinations it can make with other molecules, such as in cell membrane construction. Proper construction of the cell membrane is essential to proper function. Through evolution, our body has developed by using fats found in food. In the past 50 years or so, synthetic or altered fats have been introduced into our diets with deleterious effect. As you will read in the discussion of trans-fatty acids, it is important that we avoid synthetic fats and we should stick to the fats that Mother Nature has always supplied for us.

Plants and animals both make fats. Animals need fat for energy stores and many other uses: major components of cell membranes, hormone synthesis, and bile, temperature insulation, cushioning against trauma, electric insulation of nerves, structure of many cells such as brain cells and pancreas, and many specialized uses. Plants make fats principally for energy storage in nuts and other seeds. Fish, being cold-blooded, need fats that will not turn solid at the colder temperatures of seawater. That is why we find the unsaturated fats in fish oils, seeds, and nuts. Cows and other animals that are warm-blooded, even in cold weather, make saturated fats that require less energy for synthesis than unsaturated fats do.

Fats feel slippery and make our food taste less dry. Avocados and papaya are more slippery-feeling than potatoes, for example. Cashew nuts are commonly added for that purpose when cooking with a wok.

Diets with less than 10% fat are generally unpalatable. Fats are slower to digest and provide more than twice the calories per pound than sugars (9 Kcal/gram versus 4 Kcal/gram); therefore, they provide more energy over a longer duration than sugars or starches. Eskimos, whose diets are full of fat (fish oils, etc.) can go a long time between meals.

Fats, unlike simple sugars, are not absorbed in the stomach. They require emulsification with bile and the pancreatic enzyme, lipase, and are absorbed principally by the small intestine into the portal vein, which carries them to the liver. They are then converted to triglyceride or cholesterol before their release into the bloodstream for transport elsewhere in the body.

Some very tiny bits of emulsified fat are absorbed directly into the blood stream as chylomicrons. These minute bits of fat wafting in the blood stream are often overlooked as a danger to health. However, this is an error. Red blood cells (RBCs), as living individual cells, generate a positive electromagnetic charge. Each rbc generates the same charge and, since like charges repel each other, the rbcs are not prone to clump together but float evenly distributed throughout blood plasma. Chylomicrons have the ability to temporarily "soak up" the rbc's electromagnetic charge which allows individual cells to clump together in a "rouleau" formation (i.e., like a stack of poker chips). Our blood vessel capillaries are so tiny that rbcs travel through them only one at a time. When a clump of packed rbcs arrive at a capillary, they cannot pass through. Thus, shortly after eating a high fat meal, blood flow through capillaries is blocked and the risk of stroke, for instance, is increased. Hippocrates (circa 400 BC) noted this association of stroke after a high fat meal.

When sugar is not sufficiently available for energy requirements, fat is mobilized from fat storage sites for transportation to muscle cells where they can be metabolized as fuel. Since they lack the oxygen atoms of sugar molecules, this metabolism requires a much greater oxygen supply by the cells using them. When oxygen demand is being met during exercise, it is called "aerobic." Without sufficient oxygen, fats can not be used efficiently for fuel (and toxic compounds result) and the muscle cells must rely on sugar if it is available at the time.

Certain special fats made by plants are essential (i.e., we would die for lack of them) to humans. Vitamin E, an important antioxidant, is one such special fat. Vitamin A, another fat-soluble vitamin, is made by animals, usually from betacarotene provided by plants. Vitamin D is also fat-soluble but not found in plants. We (and other mammals) make that ourselves by converting the cholesterol precursor, cholestadienol, into vitamin D in our skin under exposure to sunshine. Now that we wear more clothes and live indoors, it is wise to supplement vitamin D in our diet. Once provided as cod liver oil, it is now routinely added to milk. As we age, however, we lose the ability to digest milk properly. Most people over 60 years of age should take a vitamin D supplement or get a 20-minute sunbath every day.

Other essential fats are the three monounsaturated fatty acids known as Omega-3, Omega-6, and Omega-9. These will be discussed more in chapter 9.

THE FAT PROBLEM OF "FEED LOT" BEEF

Time was when beef cattle were range-fed on the hoof in large acreage of grass lands. Their muscles accumulated oleic acid (a "good" fatty acid) for energy storage. Beef was a highly prized dinner item. Modern beef production now uses castrated steers penned within tightly packed feed lots, fed sorghum (high-sugar waste from sugar mills) and grain (contaminated with pesticide), and liberally dosed with estrogen (stilbestrol), the purpose of which is to increase their fat and water content to speed their getting to market weight. The muscles of these animals accumulate not oleic acid but stearic acid fat. The meat, now well-marbled with the wrong fat and loaded with fat-soluble pesticide, should no longer be a prized dinner item: stearic acid fat promotes elevated cholesterol and especially LDL cholesterol in those who eat it, and the pesticide content increases one's cancer risk.

The estrogen dosing and pesticide contamination of feed-lot beef are related. Feed-lot steers (castrated to remove testosterone) are given estrogen to promote more rapid growth and higher fat content, as mentioned above. The grain that is fed to them is heavily contaminated with pesticides of many kinds. These pesticides are petrochemical compounds that are toxic, fat-soluble, and non-biodegradable. In all animals, these drugs are hormone and endocrine disruptors. They are known as xeno (foreign) estrogens (since many of them are potent estrogens), xenohormones, or xenobiotics. They will be discussed more thoroughly in later chapters.

It is important, however, to know that British and European markets do not buy US beef because they don't want humans to be exposed to these xenohormones. One of them, 17 β-estradiol, is banned by the European Union Scientific Committee on Veterinary Medicine since it is considered a "complete carcinogen . . . [that] exerts both tumor initiating and tumor promoting effects." Even at very low levels of exposure, these xenohormones are especially potent in damaging the embryos of animals including humans, leading to abnormalities of the ovaries, testes, and other urogenital organs. One of their potential effect is to increase the risk of cancer of the breast, uterus, or prostate later in life. These hormone disruptors are used as "growth hormones" in pork and poultry, also. Since the toxic effects of these xenohormones is most potent during embryo life, it is especially important for pregnant women to choose organically (hormone-free) grown beef, chicken, or poultry in their diet.

Further, this practice of growing "feed lot" beef is environmentally unsound. Large areas of the arid US southwest, where the practice is primarily located, are devoted to growing corn and other line crops for the steers' feed, requiring extensive irrigation. The vast amounts of water used in this process not only increases the siltation loss of the available top soil but uses up about 50% of the total potable water consumed annually in the US; and is drawing down water from the underground aquifer at an alarming rate. The caloric value of the meat eventually produced represents less than 1/15 of that of the grains consumed by steers. Our continued dependence on meat such as produced in this process is not only unhealthful to us but also damaging to our precious environment.

FAT PROCESSING - THE "CIS" AND "TRANS" FORMS

Various grains and seeds are processed to extract their fats; we see them as oils sold in our food markets. They are used in the preparation of fried foods, in bakery goods, salad oils, margarine, and many other foods. They are the oils we see advertised as being derived from safflower seeds, corn, sunflower seeds, cotton seeds, palm oil, coconut oil, olive oil, rape seed oil (canola oil), and others. However, what is not generally realized is that the processed fats are not identical to oils from which they were derived. The processing by high pressure pressing, partial hydrogenation, and clarification actually changes their molecular configuration. The change in molecular shape has physiological consequences in our metabolism. Our metabolic processes have adapted to utilize food oils as found in their natural state, called *cis*-fatty acids. Such biochemical processes are dependent on the precise configuration of the molecules being metabolized. In commercial processing, fat molecules emerge in altered forms called *trans*-fatty acids. They no longer "fit" in the biochemical machinery of our metabolism and, as such, are physiologically dysfunctional and a risk to health. A good book for information on this subject is *Fats That Heal, Fats That Kill* by Udo Erasmus, a paperback published by alive books, 1994. Flaxseed oil and olive oil require less pressure in pressing and thus remain in their natural state. Flaxseed oil, however, is more likely to oxidize (go rancid) when exposed to light or air.

Fat molecules are primary constituents of cell membranes, for example, and are involved with many other physiologic processes throughout the body. The use of the trans-fatty acids potentially results in deterioration of cell membranes, a greater risk of cancer and cardiovascular disease, and a degradation of one's immune system among other problems.

For over a decade, responsible scientists have pressed the FDA for a regulation requiring the identification of the concentrations of trans-fatty acids in the processed foods that are sold to us. This is now the practice in Canada but in the US the FDA has yet to act. At the present time, our choices of fats and oils should follow the list below.

GOOD FATS (cis-fatty acids)	BAD FATS (trans-fatty acids)
Fish and seafood oils	Homogenized milk fats
Flaxseed oil	Processed oils
Olive oil	Tropical oils (e.g., palm oil)
Canola oil (probably)	Feed lot beef
Eggs are OK	Margarine
A little butter is OK	Cottonseed oils

SOURCES OF FAT: AN EXAMPLE

Dietary sources and the quantities of fat ingested are often not recognized or easily quantified in normal, every day food choices. This is particularly true of food prepared by "fast food" restaurants, as the list below demonstrates.

FOOD	CALORIES	FAT (G)	CALORIES FROM FAT	PERCENT CALORIES
McDonald's				
McLean Deluxe sandwich	320	10	90	28.1%
Filet-O-Fish sandwich	440	26	234	53.2%
McLean Deluxe, French fries	540	22	198	36.7%
Biscuit w/Sausage & Egg	529	35	315	59.5%
Burger King				
BK Broiler Chicken sandwich	379	13	117	30.9%
Double Whopper w/cheese	935	61	549	58.7%
Croissan'wich w/Sausage	538	41	366	68.0%
Wendy's				
Grilled Chicken sandwich	340	13	117	34.4%
Wendy's Big Classic	570	33	297	52.1%
Triple Cheeseburger	1,040	68	614	59.0%

FOOD CONTINUED...	CALORIES	FAT (G)	CALORIES FROM FAT	PERCENT CALORIES
Kentucky Fried Chicken				
Lite 'n Crispy Drumsticks	242	14	162	52.1%
Chicken sandwich	482	27	243	50.4%
Hardee's				
Oat Bran Muffin	440	18	162	36.8%
Real Lean Deluxe, small fries	577	25	221	38.4%
Big Deluxe, small fries	730	41	369	50.6%
Big Country Breakfast (Sausage)	1,005	74	663	66.0%

Source: Nutrition Action Newsletter, September 1989

In above example, not only is the fat content high, but the fats are likely to be trans-fatty acids. Even if a restaurant uses "good" oils for its deep-fat frying, the longer the oil is heated, the more likely it is to become oxidized (rancid) over time.

HUMAN SYNTHESIS OF FAT

It is a mistake to think that our body fat comes strictly from the fat we eat. Like all animals, we make fat from carbohydrates – sugars, starches, and complex carbohydrates of all sorts. In fact, the major portion of our body fat comes from dietary carbohydrates, especially sugar and refined starches. As described in the previous chapter, all the sugar and starch we eat that is not burned for energy is converted into fat. Anything that stimulates insulin will increase fat storage since insulin not only converts sugar into fat but also prevents the body from using stored body fat for energy. The more highly glycemic carbohydrates we eat, the fatter we become. Dietary fat, on the other hand, stimulates body tissues to utilize fat for energy. Diets that are low in fat and protein and high in carbohydrates will always fail to promote meaningful weight loss, regardless of calorie intake.

THE CHOLESTEROL "PROBLEM"

Cholesterol, strictly speaking, is not a fat but a special alcohol wax with many of the characteristics of fats, i.e., it dissolves well in fats but poorly in water. To biochemists, the word "sterol" means "ring-shaped"; the "chole" part refers to bile. Cholesterol is a major ingredient in bile; thus its name. No plant makes cholesterol. All animals make cholesterol; its major site of synthesis in humans is the liver. It is made primarily from sugar and other starches, and less from fats. The carbon atoms are linked together in 6-carbon chains which are eventually joined in such a way that four rings are made into a special formation pictured below.

The Cholesterol Molecule

Cholesterol has many functions: brain cells need it; it is an efficient method of energy storage; it is an important constituent of cell membranes and nerve sheath (myelin) insulation; and (very important) it is necessary for the synthesis of vitamin D and all our steroid hormones such as cortisone and the gonadal hormones (progesterone, testosterone and estrogen). After synthesis in the liver, cholesterol is enveloped in a protein for transport through the bloodstream. It accumulates at the site of inflamed lining cells of our arteries but its usual target is a fat cell (for storage) or an organ that needs it for further use as a precursor for the synthesis of important hormones.

When enveloped in its protein covering, the cholesterol is called a lipo-protein and it is in that form that it circulates through the blood stream. There are two slightly different types. One is nicely soluble in blood and is called "high density lipo-protein," or HDL, and the other is not so soluble in blood and is called "low density lipo-protein," or LDL, because it tends to separate and float at the top of a blood sample. The HDL cholesterol is referred to as the "good" cholesterol because it does not clog up arteries; LDL cholesterol is considered the "bad" cholesterol because it is more susceptible to oxidation (i.e., becoming rancid) and is the one that can clog up arteries.

The total and relative amounts of these two cholesterol compounds are determined in part by genetics and part by diet and exercise. It is better, of course, to have as high a ratio as possible of the HDL variety, relative to total cholesterol. Differences in HDL and LDL levels are due to several factors of which genetics, diet, and exercise are the most important. Since one's genetics can not be changed, one must concentrate on diet and exercise. In general, excess intake of starches and fats (above those needed for energy and repair processes) will put on weight, raise total cholesterol, and increase the LDL fraction. In this regard, dietary sugar and refined starches are more potent than dietary fat in raising LDL-cholesterol and triglyceride concentrations. (ref. *Lancet* 1999; 353: 1045-48) Further, not all fats are the same in regard to cholesterol. Intake of certain fats (see below) will raise the LDL ratio, other fats will favor the HDL ratio. It is important to avoid the LDL-raising fats and favor the HDL-raising fats. Aerobic exercise tends to lower total cholesterol and raise the HDL ratio, and thus is especially beneficial in this regard.

A listing of the HDL-raising and LDL-raising fats follows:

HDL-raising Fats	LDL-raising Fats
Fish oils (salmon, cod, etc.)	"Jungle" fats (coconut & palm oil)
Vegetable oils (fresh state)	Dairy fats, esp. homogenized milk
Olive oil	"Feedlot" fats (most red meat)
Eggs are fine	Pressed grain or nut oils
Shell fish foods are fine	Hydrogenated oils of any kind (e.g., margarine)
Free range animal fat	

Notice that this list is essentially identical to the list of cis- and trans=form fats. Also note that egg yolks are no longer considered to be bad, regardless of their cholesterol content. (ref. *JAMA* 1999; 281: 1387-1394) There is no study that shows a cholesterol-raising risk from egg eating, just as there is no study that shows a risk of heart disease from egg eating. It is simplistic and wrong to think that eating egg yolks will raise one's cholesterol, just as it is wrong to think that eating hair will increase the hair on one's head.

Elevated cholesterol levels are associated with the development of atherosclerosis, i.e., the accumulation of fatty substances within our arteries. This will impair blood flow and can lead to heart attacks and strokes. HDL cholesterol has the ability to "pick up" LDL cholesterol and carry it back to the liver where it can be excreted in bile. Furthermore, HDL is more resistant to oxidation than is LDL. It is the oxidation of cholesterol that most probably leads to atherosclerosis. (See chapter 9.) Thus, HDL cholesterol protects us from strokes and heart attacks. Also, antioxidants vitamins C and E protect against oxidation of cholesterol and thereby protect us from heart attacks.

The "total" cholesterol level in our blood is, except for the extreme ranges, not a good indicator of this cardiovascular risk. The great majority of people with heart attacks have total cholesterol levels in the normal range. When serum cholesterol is measured, it is important to also measure the HDL fraction. The ratio of HDL-cholesterol to total cholesterol is a far better predictor of heart attacks. In the US, the average ratio of HDL to total cholesterol is 1:5, or 20%. The average in the US. is not especially healthy, as the US leads the world in the incidence of heart attack deaths. It would be much better if the HDL: total cholesterol ratio were 1:3 or 33% HDL, for example. These relationships will be more thoroughly discussed in chapter 9.

Cholesterol vignette #1.

A healthy looking 65-year old woman came to see me about her cholesterol problem. For years she had been found to have a high total cholesterol level (300 mg/dl) and she was concerned about the possibility of heart disease. She played tennis regularly, felt fine, and ate a good diet. Her previous doctors had been very concerned about her cholesterol but nothing they did had changed it. I repeated her blood tests and found that, while her total cholesterol reading was 300, her HDL-cholesterol was 110 mg/dl. After explaining the significance of the good ratio and assuring her she had no reason to change her diet, I asked her why she had come to see me instead of her previous doctors. She told me they had all died of heart attacks: she had outlived her doctors. I told her she might also outlive me. She is now in her late 80s and doing fine.

Cholesterol vignette #2.

Not far from my office was a grocery store in which a slim 50-year old man worked. He, knowing I was a doctor, occasionally talked with me about medical things. One day he quite proudly told me his cholesterol level was 180. The next time I was in the store, another worker told me our friend was in the hospital with a heart attack. I visited him in the hospital and, by chance, happened to talk with his doctor. I inquired about his cholesterol levels and learned that his total cholesterol was indeed 180 or so but his HDL-cholesterol was only 10. His ratio of HDL- to total cholesterol was 1:18! That is a very bad ratio, despite his low total cholesterol. Sometimes, the Fates provide a little lesson when we least expect it.

Conventional "wisdom" thinks that eating fat, especially cholesterol-rich food, causes serum cholesterol concentrations to rise, and the serum cholesterol is the cause of atherosclerosis. Neither of these are true. Sugar and refined carbohydrates are more potent than fat in raising serum cholesterol, a discovery brought to our attention over 30 years ago by Dr. John Yudkin of England, and reaffirmed recently by Frost, Leeds, Dore et al in *Lancet* 1999; 353: 1045-48. And cholesterol, per se, is not the *cause* of atherosclerosis; it is a marker of a underlying disorder wrought by metabolic imbalance. This will be discussed more thoroughly in chapter 9.

THE GOOD EGG?

Is there really a clear relationship between blood cholesterol level/coronary heart disease and the number of eggs we eat? Apparently not, according to data from the Boston University-Framingham Heart Study, which has been investigating heart-risk factors for more than 25 years. Comparing egg intakes of 912 Framingham, Massachusetts, residents, researchers found no evidence of any significant association between egg consumption and deaths from coronary heart disease: nor was there any notable association between eggs and heart attack or angina pectoris (the chest pain associated with heart disease). In addition, Dr. Thomas R. Dawber and his co-workers found no marked differences in the actual blood cholesterol levels between subjects who ate many eggs per week (7 to 24) and those who ate few (0 to 2.5).

Reported by *Boston University Medical Center Centerscope* 1990;14:6

The notion that egg yolks raise serum cholesterol levels because they contain cholesterol is a fixture of the present cholesterol fallacy. The simple fact is there is no human study that shows this to be the case. In *JAMA* (1999; 281: 1387-94), a review of the Health Professionals Follow-up Study (1986-1994) found no evidence of an association between egg consumption (from 1 egg/week to >1 egg/day) and the risk of coronary heart disease (CHD) or stroke in either men or women (except possibly in diabetes). It is time to recognize that eating cholesterol, per se, does not cause heart disease or strokes.

SUMMARY

The present fear of eating any fat or oil is unwarranted. When applied to children's diet, avoidance of fat can be damaging; it leads to poor brain development, for example. What is important is to understand the difference between "bad" fat and "good" fat. There are three categories of bad fats:

1. those that shift the balance of lipoproteins from HDL- to LDL-cholesterol

2. those that have been altered by processing into trans-fatty acids, and

3. those that are contaminated with synthetic estrogen (e.g., diethylstilbestrol [DES]) or petrochemical toxins known as xenohormones such as pesticides in feed grain.

Good fats are the naturally-occurring fats and oils in grain, seeds, nuts, and vegetables, and fats and oils from uncontaminated fish, lamb and other meat.

SELF-QUIZ

1. Saturated fat raises your blood cholesterol. True or False?

2. All unsaturated fats are nutritionally good. True or False?

3. Dietary cholesterol is the principal cause of blood cholesterol. True or False?

4. Total serum cholesterol is a good indicator of heart disease risk. True or False?

5. All animals synthesize cholesterol from starches. True or False?

6. Cholesterol is essential for many body functions. True or False?

7. Cholesterol is necessary for hormone synthesis. True or False?

8. Some plant foods are high in cholesterol. True or False?

9. The "good" cholesterol is _____ and the "bad" cholesterol is _____ .

10. The better unsaturated fats come from fish and seeds. True or False?

Answers on page 85.

CHAPTER FOUR
PROTEINS

Proteins are very large organic molecules composed of amino acids that, in addition to carbon, hydrogen, and oxygen, also contain nitrogen. A typical protein molecule is 1000 to one million times larger than a molecule of glucose, for example. Meat, fish, cheese, and egg whites are examples of protein-rich food. Good protein is also found in beans, soy and legumes. Proteins are composed of amino acids; these are rather small molecular chains in which the terminal carbon carries an oxygen and a hydroxyl radical (thus, an *organic acid*) and the penultimate (second to last) carbon is linked to an amine group (nitrogen with two hydrogens); thus the name amino acid.

| Leucine | Methionine | Phenylalanine |

There are 22 amino acids we use as building blocks to make up our proteins; they are essential for the synthesis of tissue (e.g., muscle, skin, cartilage, hair etc.), hormones, enzymes, neurotransmitters, and much more. We have the ability to convert one amino acid into another for all but eight of these 22. Those eight "essential" amino acids must be made by another animal or plant and must be in our diet for us to survive. All essential amino acids are found in meat, fish, milk, egg white and soy beans. Other foods may be deficient in one or another of the amino acids but several different foods can be combined in one's diet to supply all the essential amino acids; these are then called "complementary" foods. An example would be beans and corn; each lacks a different essential amino acid but, together, they are complete.

Essential amino acids	Other amino acids
Isoleucine	Alanine
Leucine	Arginine
Lysine	Asparagine
Methionine	Aspartic acid
Phenylalanine	Cysteine
Threonine	Hydroxylysine
Tryptophan	Hydroxyproline
Valine	Proline
	Serine
	Tyrosine
	Glutamic acid
	Glutamine
	Glycine
	Histidine

DIGESTION OF DIETARY PROTEIN

Dietary proteins must be broken down to their amino acid components. This is accomplished step-wise by pepsin and hydrochloric acid in the stomach followed by pancreatic enzymes (trypsin and chymotrypsin) and intestinal exopeptidase. If any amino acid complexes escape this arsenal of digestive enzymes, the intestinal mucosa (lining cells of the intestine) excrete dipeptidase enzymes that finish off the process of converting all protein into simple amino acids. Since digestive enzymes are proteins, it is somewhat ironic but not surprising that some digestion of these enzymes themselves does occur. This is one of the factors in creating a need for good protein intake.

While it is well established that the small intestine is capable of absorbing all amino acids, it is also known that, in some people and in some circumstances, absorption of dipeptides (small protein complexes) can also occur. This is found in a rare genetic disease known as Hartnup's disease, for example. It is also established that conditions in which the mucosal lining of the intestine is damaged by disease (prolonged oral antibiotic courses, high stress or cortisol medication, oral fluoride dosages, or severe dehydration) may lead to intestinal permeability ("leaky gut syndrome"). In these cases, patches of mucosa are denuded and absorption of incompletely digested proteins into the underlying vascular bed may take place. These protein complexes are carried in the bloodstream throughout the body. When they arrive at a capillary bed in some tissue in the body, they react as foreign bodies, causing inflammation, asthma, or pain. Supplemental antioxidants and rather large doses of the amino acid L-glutamine (500 mg several times a day) usually result in eventual healing of the gut if the offending causes can be adequately avoided.

DAILY PROTEIN INTAKE

Proteins are used for growth and repair; they are not, except in very unusual circumstances, used as fuel for energy. They make up our muscle and connective tissue (collagen fibers) e.g., tendons, cartilage, and ligaments, our enzymes, the peptides of neuro-transmitters, and the nucleic acids of our DNA . Once we reach full growth, our intake need not be very large, usually only 1.5-2.5 oz. a day. Protein-rich food such as lean meat or cheese contain 25% protein by weight. For example, 4 ounces of lean meat or cheese provides 1 oz of protein. Beans and some nuts contain 10-12% protein. Our daily protein requirement is easily met by eating meat but can also be accomplished by a good, broad-based vegetarian diet eaten in sufficient amounts. Unfortunately, the standard American diet provides 5-6 oz/day of protein. Eating more protein than we need will not help us as we have no means of storing it.

Excreting excess protein creates problems for our kidneys: amines are excreted as ammonia, and protein waste products are acids that may cause metabolic acidosis that leads to urinary calcium loss and, thus, osteoporosis. Meat, beans and cheese proteins are rich in purines, which are converted to uric acid for excretion in urine. If excretion is not efficient, the result is gout. Unabsorbed dietary proteins in our colon are fermented by colon bacteria into cancer-causing nitrosamine. It is wise, therefore, to limit protein intake. By the same token, the fact that we do not store excess protein means that it is wise to obtain sufficient protein daily. If protein intake is deficient, muscle mass decreases and brain function is impaired.

PROTEIN BIOCHEMISTRY

Amino acids have an extraordinary ability to link to one another by way of sharing hydrogen bonds and thus are used by the body to create a wide variety of different and very useful compounds in our bodies. For example, they are the building blocks of all enzymes. Enzymes are the biochemical catalysts for all life processes. Their actions result from (1) their specific molecular conformation (similar to special keys for special locks), and (2) their ability to temporarily pick up or let go of electromagnetically "charged" particles such as electrons or hydrogen ions. Amino acids are the building blocks for all protein tissues and for enzymes that are the facilitators of all life processes.

An average cell may contain over 2000 types of enzymes, each represented by millions of these macromolecules. All of them are created by special protein messengers (RNA) serving as templates derived from nuclear chromosomal and mitochondrial DNA. Though each cell has a full complement of chromosomal DNA, different cells have different functions and each prepares only the enzymes it needs to fulfill those functions. The complexity and specificity of the molecular transformations in each and every body cell is truly beyond comprehension. Anything that disturbs the synthesis and action of enzymes (such as fluoride) will be toxic in one way or another.

In addition to forming the structural material of cells and tissues, and all the enzymes needed by our body, proteins also play a pivotal role as plasma proteins (that create the osmotic pressure that maintains the watery component of blood), antibodies, hemoglobin, and certain hormones (such as insulin).

THE EXAMPLE OF TRYPTOPHAN

Earlier in this century, a terrible disease causing over 20,000 deaths developed in southern US states where corn was the major food crop for many. The disease, pellagra, was characterized by the four Ds; dermatitis, diarrhea, dementia, and death, with a wide range in the severity of the symptoms. It was eventually found to respond to niacin, one of the B vitamins. However, the problem was traced to the dependence on corn as one's main food. Corn is deficient in both niacin and the amino acid tryptophan. Subsequent research has shown that tryptophan can be converted by the body into niacin. Despite the deficiency in niacin, if corn had provided tryptophan, pellagra would not have occurred.

Tryptophan is found in abundance in mother's milk and is considered to be not only essential for growth but also is the ingredient in breast milk that leads to pacifying the child and causing sleepiness. (Another good source is dark turkey meat.) This ability to induce sleep has been found especially important in the treatment of alcoholic patients where it is safely and effectively used as a sedative which, unlike most barbiturates and other sedatives, does not impose a burden on the liver.

In 1989, a strange disease characterized by severe muscle pains and an elevation of eosinophilic blood cells (thus called eosinophilia-myalgia syndrome) developed. The disease was traced to the use of tryptophan supplements made by the Showa Denka pharmaceutical company of Japan and the FDA quickly banned the use of all tryptophan. Tryptophan is synthesized commercially by bacterial fermentation from anthranilate followed by a complex purification process. Further research found that the production technique of this one company had allowed a toxic contaminant to be included with the tryptophan they sold which was then re-sold under different labels by different supplement providers here in the US. Shortly thereafter, the production problem was corrected. When subsequent research showed no trace of the contaminant in any tryptophan being sold, countries around the world resumed the therapeutic use of tryptophan. In the US, however, the FDA at this date continues to prohibit the sale of over the counter tryptophan despite the fact that no medical problem is encountered elsewhere in the world where tryptophan is sold. Regardless of the political implications, this example reveals the exquisite specificity and safety of the natural compound, tryptophan, compared to the potential danger of synthetically-derived copies of the same compound.

CALCULATING PROTEIN CONTENT OF FOODS

Meats, chicken, turkey, cheese and fish are excellent sources of protein. As a general rule, 25% of meat is protein, the rest being fat, muscle glycogen, water, and ash. Thus, four ounces of hamburger will provide one ounce of protein. This is slightly less than in chicken or turkey since less fat is present in the muscles of these fowl. All of them contain a full complement of the essential amino acids.

Protein content of vegetables, legumes and nuts ranges from 3.5 - 12 %. Except for soy, plant foods lack one or another of the essential amino acids. When several are eaten together and thereby provide the full complement, they are called "complementary" foods. A vegetarian diet that consists of a wide variety of different vegetables, legumes, nuts and whole grains will not be lacking in any of the essential amino acids.

Egg white is composed of albumin and, like meat, provides all essential amino acids. The protein found in one standard egg white is 0.22 ounces, i.e., a bit over a fifth of an ounce. Recall that our optimal protein intake should be about 1.5-2.5 ounces per day. The following list will help you calculate your daily protein intake.

The protein content of various foods.

Most meats .... approximately 25% protein

Chicken, turkey, cheese and fish .... 25-30 % protein

Beans, peas, and nuts .... approximately 10-12 % protein

Other vegetables... range from 3.5-10 % protein

One egg (egg white)......................... 0.22 oz of protein (same as one bagel)

CONSEQUENCES OF SEVERE PROTEIN DEFICIENCY

The importance of adequate protein intake can not be overemphasized. Protein deficiency results in complex pathological changes. In the young, protein deficiency characteristically causes growth to stop. In both the young and old, bones become rarefied, cell proliferation is depressed, collagen formation in connective tissue is much reduced, skin atrophies, hair and fingernails are lost, muscles atrophy, the liver loses function, neurotransmitters in the brain and nervous system malfunction, and digestion function is lost. Death is the ultimate consequence.

Serious protein deficiency in young children leads to skinny hollow-eyed kids with bulging abdomens. The bulging abdomens result from weakness of abdominal muscles. This condition is known as *kwashiorkor.* Afflicted children show signs of edema, mental changes, and fatty infiltration of the liver. If combined with energy deficiency (starvation), the condition is called *marasmus.* Examples can be found in many Third World countries.

PROTEINS AND THE MEANING OF LIFE

Living things are energetic; they utilize, transform, and create energy in ways not found in non-living things. Green plants contain chlorophyll (a protein compound containing magnesium) to utilize solar energy to transform carbon dioxide (CO_2) and water (H_2O) into carbohydrates. Our bodies use carbohydrates and transform them into glucose and fats essential for our lives. We use a compound similar to chlorophyll, called hemoglobin, which is also a protein compound but containing iron, to carry oxygen throughout the body. We use the oxygen to "oxidize" fuel such as glucose and fat into energy for muscles, brain power, and all the biochemical action our body needs.

When wood is oxidized (burned) in a stove, heat and light energy are obtained. This is oxidation on a massive scale. Our body's way of oxidizing our fuel is different; it takes place on a submicroscopic scale by millions of tiny steps we call metabolism. The mechanism is electromagnetic, transferring electrons from one compound to another using ions of H, OH, and phosphorous (P). The life force of animal life is electromagnetism. It oxidizes fuel for the energy of our cells without producing much heat or light. Since our cells can only live within a rather limited temperature range, excessive heat production (like burning wood) would kill them. Electromagnetism is the key to transferring energy in minute steps with great efficiency but without much heat. If a watermelon were dropped from a 10-story building, it would accumulate considerable kinetic energy and splatter to pieces when it hit the ground. Our electromagnetic system is more like walking down the stairs one step at a time, using the kinetic energy in many little steps so as to be not damaged in the process.

Ancient philosophers gave the metaphysical name, "Chi," to life energy. This is roughly translatable as electromagnetic energy. In this process, the key performer is protein. Amino acids (building blocks of protein) have the remarkable capacity to carry, transfer, and modulate the oxidizing of chemical bonds to obtain energy and perform the electromagnetic magic of our metabolic systems. If we fail to provide the essential protein and co-factors for these systems, or block its function in any way, our "Chi" weakens and our health suffers. When we run out of "Chi," we die.

Thus, protein, more than any other dietary component, is the key to life itself.

SELF QUIZ

1. Proteins are composed of amino acids. True or False?

2. All meat contains all essential amino acids. True or False?

3. All vegetables contain all essential amino acids. True or False?

4. In general, vegetarian diets include all essential amino acids. True or False?

5. In typical adults, daily protein intake should be only 1.5-2 oz/day. True or False?

6. Proteins are good for providing energy. True or False?

7. Eating more protein than is necessary does no harm. True or False?

8. All proteins include carbon, hydrogen, oxygen and
   _____.

9. The protein in eggs is in the yolks. True or False?

10. Excess dietary protein can cause osteoporosis. True or False?

Answers can be found on page 85.

CHAPTER FIVE
MINERALS, VITAMINS, MICRONUTRIENTS AND FIBER

MINERALS

Minerals are those elements we associate with rocks and soil where they combine to make crystalline hard compounds. Minerals become incorporated in bone but every cell in our body uses them and contains them just as every drop of water in the ocean has a certain amount of dissolved minerals. In nutritional science, they are divided into "major" (daily intake 1 gram or more) and "minor" (daily intake less than 1 gram) minerals. The major minerals are calcium, chloride, potassium, magnesium, sodium, and phosphorous. The minor minerals are boron, cobalt, chromium, copper, iron, iodine, manganese, molybdenum, selenium, silicon, and zinc (and probably others in trace amounts).

Minerals are used for building body structures (e.g., calcium in bones) and, when dissolved and in ionic form (i.e., electrolytes), as catalysts for biochemical processes. All biological processes are dependent on enzymes; all enzyme action requires vitamins and minerals as catalysts. Therefore, intake of minerals is truly essential. The same is true for plants. Eating plants, therefore, is a good way of acquiring minerals. Most minerals are, to different degrees, soluble in water and are dissolved out of plants when they are cooked in water. Therefore, plants should be eaten without prolonged cooking in water or, if they are, the water should be drunk as in soups & stews. Many canned and frozen vegetables have been cooked in water and the water discarded prior to canning; thus they are not as good a source of minerals as are fresh vegetables. Minerals are not destroyed by cooking; they have merely transferred to the water, which was discarded. Microwave cooking does not damage the minerals in food.

POTASSIUM/SODIUM

Certain minerals must be supplied in amounts that relate to that of other minerals. This is true of calcium to magnesium, calcium to phosphorous, and sodium to potassium, for example. Consider the potassium/sodium problem in our modern diets. All unrefined foods provide potassium and sodium in a ratio of 20-200 parts potassium to 1 part sodium. We have, throughout history, been supplied with abundant potassium and very little sodium. We therefore have developed good mechanisms for excreting excess potassium in urine but not for sodium. To obtain sufficient sodium, animals (and man) developed a salt "taste" for seeking out extra sodium. The benefits of a little extra sodium (salt or "sal") are reflected in our words "salutation," "salary," and "salubrious."

Our cells are surrounded by water. Potassium and magnesium are the dominant electrolytes within cells (intracellular fluid) and sodium is the dominant electrolyte in the water outside of cells (extracellular fluid). Since the membrane enclosing each cell is a semipermeable membrane, there is something of a mystery about how this separation of mineral electrolytes comes about. If the membrane were only a passive membrane, the concentrations of minerals within and outside the cell would be the same. The cell membrane, however, is a living, active structure with the capability to maintain magnesium and potassium within the cell, and keep the sodium outside in the extracellular fluid. This ability is called a pump.

These pumps perform well when our intake of potassium and sodium matches that of natural foods. In processed foods, much mineral content has been lost and the food lacks flavor. The food processors add sodium chloride to the foods to give them a "zesty" taste. This processing reverses the ratios of potassium and magnesium to sodium so that, for example, for every one part potassium we may now have 200 to 1200 parts sodium. Our cells are incapable of handling this imbalance. The excess sodium attracts excess water; and intracellular potassium and magnesium concentrations can not be maintained. Our cell action deteriorates, our bodies fill with water. The body attempts to rid itself of excess sodium by increasing the pressure of the blood flow into the kidney to force out more water. Doctors call this "essential" hypertension. (See chapter 10)

It is important to realize that the sodium from our processed foods often reaches a total of 8-10,000 mg/day. In areas of the world where processed foods are uncommon, hypertension is rare. Even dietitians may be unaware of the sodium imbalance in canned foods, cereals, baked goods (sodium bicarbonate), etc. Of course, salt has long been used as a food preservative (e.g., salt pork) but that is usually a minor component of the total diet and probably needed to replace the sodium lost, those days, in the sweat of manual labor. A daily intake of 1500-3000 mg of sodium is usually adequate.

PHOSPHORUS/CALCIUM

Another example is the phosphorus/calcium ratio. Homeostasis demands that the serum concentrations of calcium and phosphorus are held to a specific ratio. If phosphorus intake increases and calcium intake does not, calcium will be leached out of bone to restore the proper ratio. Foods containing relatively high levels of phosphorus but lacking in calcium are red meat and artificially carbonated beverages (once called "phospho-sodas"). Milk products such as cheese contain both calcium and phosphorus and thus are beneficial during childhood when bone growth is active.

(Milk, however, lacks sufficient magnesium that is necessary for calcium incorporation into bone. Therefore, it is wise to make sure that one's magnesium intake from other sources is adequate. See below.)

CALCIUM

Let us briefly consider another calcium example. The great majority (99%) of calcium in our bodies is found in bones. Since bones are continually being made, un-made, and made anew throughout life, there is a constant need for calcium intake of at least 600 milligrams (1/50th of an oz) per day. Many people think the best source of calcium is from milk. But where do cows get the calcium to put in their milk? The obvious answer is - from the grass, hay, and pasturage they eat. Plants are the only organism that can extract calcium from soil and incorporate it into something animals can eat and digest. In plants, it contributes to the strength of leaves, stems, and stalks. We may not be able to digest the cellulose of these tissues but we can absorb the calcium. Spinach, chard, beet tops, Chinese cabbage, and other broad leaf vegetables are excellent sources of calcium. A cup of these vegetables provides as much calcium as a cup of milk (300 mg). Some of these plants (e.g., spinach) also contain phytic and oxalic acids, which are said to interfere with calcium absorption. The degree of interference, however, is not great and generally can be ignored.

We need hydrochloric acid and vitamin D to absorb calcium. Older folks tend to make less hydrochloric acid; they also lose the ability to digest milk properly. Therefore, calcium intake and absorption becomes a little tricky with age. The answer is to supplement with vitamin D and also with hydrochloric acid (HCl) if gastric HCl production is deficient. Calcium citrate is somewhat better absorbed than other calcium products when gastric hydrochloric acid is low. To avoid dairy fats, we can use skim milk cheese along with the vegetables. It is not difficult to obtain sufficient calcium throughout all of life. If insurance is desired, a supplement of 300 mg of calcium and 150 mg of magnesium can be used.

MAGNESIUM
Second only to potassium, magnesium is an intracellular mineral electrolyte of major importance. Though the body's need for magnesium is less than sodium, potassium or calcium, it serves as a catalyst for more enzymes than any other mineral. It functions as a co-catalyst with the B vitamins for many enzymes and, as such, it facilitates the proper utilization of these vitamins. Magnesium is a relaxant for smooth muscles; thus it is effective in preventing arterial contraction such as occurs in angina and the hypertension of preeclampsia (toxemia of pregnancy - headache, hypertension, retinal hemorrhages, nausea and vomiting, edema, proteinuria, and oliguria) and eclampsia (the development of convulsions and coma).

Magnesium helps the body absorb and utilize calcium. If magnesium levels are low, high calcium intake leads to elevated serum calcium with the result that secretion of calcitonin increases and parathyroid hormone is suppressed. In this event, calcium is not deposited in bones but, instead, is deposited abnormally in soft tissues, leading to the paradox of simultaneous osteoporosis and excess soft tissue and periarticular calcifications such as are found in arthritis. With adequate magnesium, bones receive the calcium and the soft tissues do not. Magnesium has been found to be effective in relieving PMS (premenstrual syndrome), probably because it helps block undesirable side effects of excess estrogen.

Of crucial importance is the benefit of magnesium in decreasing the risk of death due to myocardial infarction. During a heart attack, coronary arteries can go into spasm (reducing the flow of blood to the heart muscle at risk) and arrhythmia is common: both can be lethal and both occur more commonly when magnesium is deficient. Magnesium given intravenously at the time of a heart attack can be life-saving. Alcoholics are especially prone to develop cardiomyopathy (a pathologic condition of the heart muscle) secondary to hypomagnesia (low magnesium levels) which leads to heart failure and death.

How does one prevent magnesium deficiency? Begin with a magnesium-rich diet. Magnesium is found in whole grains (brown rice, millet, buckwheat, whole wheat, triticale, quinoa, and rye) as well as legumes (lentils, split peas, and all varieties of beans). Essentially all fresh vegetables contain not only magnesium but the other important minerals as well. Cocoa powder, from which chocolate is made, is richer in magnesium than any other food. Chocolate craving may indicate a need for more magnesium. Dairy products contain nine times more calcium than magnesium, a ratio that leads to calcium excess and magnesium deficiency. Sugar and alcohol lead to urinary loss of magnesium. The protection against osteoporosis enjoyed by people on a vegetarian diet is probably due to their better intake of magnesium, more than double that of the standard American diet. Again it is evident that a diet high in fresh, unprocessed vegetables and whole grains is far superior to one of meat, mashed potatoes, sugar and milk.

The US Dept. of Agriculture warns, however, that magnesium intake has declined. This is partly due to the fact that our farming soil is becoming depleted in magnesium, and thus the plants we harvest contain less of it than they did a generation or two ago. Farmers replenish NPK (nitrogen, phosphorus, and potassium) in soil but not magnesium. Thus, magnesium deficiency is becoming common. In my opinion, it is wise to replenish our own magnesium levels by taking a daily 300mg supplement of magnesium complex.

Since magnesium is primarily an intracellular mineral, standard blood serum levels are poor indicators of one's magnesium status. A far better test is a measurement of red blood cell magnesium, and can be easily obtained.

Magnesium vignette:

A major function of magnesium in plants is its inclusion in the chlorophyll molecule activating it to be able to utilize the energy of sunshine to create carbohydrates from carbon dioxide and water, a process that releases oxygen to the air. This is the oxygen upon which animals (including man) are able to exist. Further, the energy of the sun that went into the formation of the plant carbohydrate's chemical bonds is the source of the energy we derive from eating and metabolizing food. And magnesium in the plant chlorophyll is the cause of the beautiful green color of plants that make up the major life form on Earth.

IRON

The example of iron excretion provides a good illustration of the various ways of the body's handling of different minerals, with iron being the interesting exception to the general rule. Most minerals, if taken in excess of the body's need, can be excreted promptly by the kidney. Body iron supply is controlled not by elimination in urine or feces but by its rate of absorption from the gut. Total body iron is not large; on average it amounts to about only 4 grams, the mass of a 3-inch nail. Most of it is incorporated in hemoglobin (in red blood cells) and ferritin (stored in liver and spleen). Its primary physiologic importance is as a component of hemoglobin and myoglobin (in muscle cells) but smaller amounts are found in special proteins, such as cytochromes, which are vital to normal cellular function. In the body, iron is in a dynamic state, moving rapidly from one molecule to another, due mainly to the steady catabolism (destruction) of senescent red blood cells. Each day, about 1% of our red blood cells are destroyed, releasing about 25 mg of iron, most of it conserved and re-used. The normal daily loss of iron in adult men and non-menstruating females is only about 1 mg, of which half is lost from the gastro-intestinal tract and the other half lost from skin cells shed each day. Menstruating females will lose 1.4 to 3.2 mg/day.

Iron is widely distributed in foodstuffs and one would think that a replacement of only 1-3 mg/day would be easily accomplished. However, only about 5% of dietary iron is absorbed. Iron exists in two chemical forms, ferrous (Fe^{2+}) or ferric (Fe^{3+}) form. Ferric forms are much less soluble (and less absorbable) than ferrous forms. In addition, dietary iron can be categorized into two types. One, which accounts for approximately 90% of iron from food is in the form of iron salts and is called the non-heme iron, i.e., the ferric or ferrous forms. The second, constituting 10% of dietary iron, is the heme type, derived from hemoglobin and myoglobin of meat. Heme iron is especially well absorbed.

Dietary iron is transferred into the intestinal mucosal cell by a small soluble iron-binding protein and then transferred again into the plasma by becoming bound to the iron transport protein, transferrin, or to the iron storage protein, ferritin. The body's absorption of iron is regulated by the degree of saturation of transferrin with iron. This, in turn, is a reflection of the adequacy of iron storage. If we need more iron, we will absorb it better; if we are well supplied, we absorb it poorly. How then, in the absence of excessive blood loss, does iron deficiency occur? Remember that "iron-deficiency" anemia is the leading cause of anemia.

Dietary factors play a significant role in the absorption of iron. Vitamin C (ascorbic acid) greatly enhances iron absorption and utilization. Orange juice, for example, doubles the absorption of non-heme iron, whereas tea decreases it by 75%. Heme iron itself promotes absorption of non-heme iron. Thus, adults absorb about four times as much non-heme iron from a mixed meal when the meal protein source is meat, fish, or chicken than when it is milk, cheese, or other dairy products. Milk casein binds to iron and prevents its absorption. If you are found to have "iron-deficiency" anemia, all that is usually necessary is to defer eating milk or cheese, and supplement a good dose (1-2 grams/day) of vitamin C. Within a week or two, your iron deficiency will have disappeared. Remember, the diet was probably not iron-deficient, per se, but some of your dietary choices and lack of vitamin C merely hindered iron absorption.

The converse situation exists in the genetic disease, hemochromatosis, in which iron absorption is greater than body needs due to abnormal transferrin control. Excess iron in the body is toxic; it accumulates in the liver and spleen and leads not only to liver damage but also to destruction of bones and cartilage, a higher risk of cardiovascular disease, and to cancer, especially of the liver and colon. Once thought to be rare, the carrier state of this disease (hemochromatosis) exists in about 1 of 40 in the US population. It is revealed by measurement of serum iron, total iron-binding capacity, serum ferritin and serum ferritin saturation levels. Intake of iron-rich food must be avoided by patients with this disease.

Because of their rapid growth, infants require a relatively higher intake of iron than adults do. In this regard, it is important to know that mothers' breast milk is superior to cow's milk. Though each contains about 0.5 to 1.0 mg of iron per liter, the absorption of iron from breast milk is about 50% on the average, compared to only 10% from cow's milk. Because of the differences in breast milk and cow's milk, the following guidelines should be followed in infant feeding:

1. Breast feed for five to six months at least. Longer is even better.

2. When solid foods are introduced into the diet, be sure to include an iron-enriched cereal.

3. Feeding whole cow's milk should be avoided during the first year of life because it may cause gastrointestinal bleeding.

4. If an infant is not breast fed, use an iron-fortified formula and supplement with small doses of vitamin E.

In summary, the best way to acquire the minerals our bodies need is to eat a variety of plants in a manner that preserves their minerals for eating, i.e., fresh, lightly steamed, as soups or stews, or by microwave.

VITAMINS

Vitamins are a heterogeneous group of organic compounds that are uniquely essential to human life for the purpose of regulating metabolism, energy synthesis, and to prevent destructive oxidation of cells; and, we are unable to synthesize them. One exception here; vitamin D is synthesized by skin and used in the stomach for absorption of calcium. Therefore, vitamin D is technically not a true vitamin but is, in fact, a hormone. In the past, it was supplemented (as cod liver oil) to children in northern climes during the winter because the cold requires heavy clothing that prevents sufficient skin exposure to whatever sun there is. Vitamin D is now routinely added to milk. We use vitamins as chemical catalysts, i.e., they modulate the direction and rate of chemical reactions without themselves being used up in the process. The exception to that rule is vitamin C, which functions also as an antioxidant and is destroyed in the process.

Vitamins are divided into two groups according to their solubility in water or fat. The water-soluble vitamins are the B vitamins, biotin, folic acid and vitamin C. Vitamins A, D, E, and K are fat-soluble. Vitamin B-12 is not found in plant foods (except comfrey): vegetarians in underdeveloped countries are said to receive their B-12 from insect residue in their diets or from colon bacteria. Our need for the other B vitamins is easily met by a diet rich in unprocessed foods. Vitamin E (also an antioxidant) is plentiful in vegetable oils and whole grains but, due to the generally poor diet in the US, most of us can benefit by a vitamin E supplement. Yellow and dark green vegetables also contain betacarotene, the precursor for conversion into vitamin A by all our cells. The only vitamins truly requiring supplementation beyond dietary intake are vitamin C and, possibly, vitamin D in older adults who may avoid skin exposure to sunlight. Almost all animals make vitamin C at the rate of about 4 grams per 150 lbs of body weight per day. We make none and our typical dietary intake is only 60 mg/day, or 1/70th of the usual animal's daily synthesis.

Many plants provide good amounts of vitamin C and our ancestors undoubtedly ingested 1000-2000 mg (1-2 gm) daily because they ate their foods essentially fresh and unprocessed. After being picked, many leafy plants such as cabbage or lettuce will lose 90% of their vitamin C content within 36-48 hours. If we ate our foods straight out of the garden, we would not need to supplement with vitamin C.

Assigning specific functions to specific vitamins is misleading. As mentioned above, vitamins serve as catalysts for multiple enzymes and therefore have multiple and diverse functions. A few examples of some singular actions of vitamins include the following:

— severe deficiency of thiamine (B1) leads to beriberi disease

— thiamine (B1) protects against alcohol-induced encephalopathy

— niacin (B3) deficiency (in the absence of tryptophan) leads to pellagra

— niacin facilitates mucus drainage and can aid memory in some

— niacin lowers cholesterol

— vitamin B12 deficiency is the cause of pernicious anemia

— folic acid (a B vitamin) prevents neural tube defects in newborns

— vitamin D deficiency causes rickets (inadequate bone mineralization)

— vitamin A deficiency leads to night blindness, skin and bone diseases

— vitamin C deficiency is the cause of scurvy (collagen deterioration)

— vitamin C also protects against viral illnesses, cancer, and some toxins

— vitamin C also lowers cholesterol and protects against heart attacks

— vitamin E protects against cataracts, respiratory and heart diseases

— pyroxidine (B6) with magnesium protects against carpal tunnel syndrome

In the vitamin B12 example above, it is important to know that pernicious anemia is not generally due to a deficiency of B12 intake but to a constitutional deficiency of a special glycoprotein called "intrinsic factor," a stomach-secreted substance that greatly aids B12 absorption. Without "intrinsic factor," our absorption of B12 is reduced 1000-fold. Thus, US doctors often treat pernicious anemia with monthly injections of B12. However, our daily need for B12 is only 1 mcg (microgram). In other countries (particularly Scandinavia), doctors prescribe oral B12 in doses 1000 times greater, or 1 mg daily, with success. Once thought to be unique to B12, similar specific intrinsic factors are found to be necessary for absorption of other vitamins, if not the majority of them.

Vitamin C vignette:

It is historically interesting that the anti-scurvy effect of limes and other fresh fruit was discovered by a British Naval Surgeon (Dr. James Lind) in the mid-1700s and that this discovery made the British navy considerably more effective than other navies of the time. To this day, British sailors are called "Limeys." The

US navy, on the other hand, regarded the concept as foolish because they had tested the Key lime (Caribbean-grown) and found it ineffective. They did not know that the Key lime is the only citrus fruit which does not contain vitamin C. It was not until the 1890s (over 150 years after Dr. Lind's discovery) that the US navy began systematic use of vitamin C-containing fruit. The active ingredient was finally identified by Albert Szent-Gyorgi and Charles King in the years 1928-33 when they also determined that the Hungarian red pepper is an extremely good source. Contemporary medicine in the US today still lags in its understanding of the benefits of vitamin C.

Another vitamin C vignette:

Almost all animals synthesize vitamin C, usually in the order of four grams/day or more per 150 lbs of animal. Among the very few animals that do not synthesize vitamin C are the rind-eating bat of India, the South American Rhesus monkey, the guinea pig, the parakeet, and humans. All of these animals, in ages past, chose a diet which included sufficient vitamin C and thus had no need to spend the energy to synthesize it. In more recent times, man has adopted a diet of stored and/or processed foods deficient in this valuable vitamin. Ironically, man, the one animal intellectually equipped to understand the importance of vitamin C and measure it in his food, is the only one that now chooses a diet deficient in it and ignores the need to supplement it.

Historic vitamin A vignette:

Many of the polar explorers failed in their efforts because they did not know that the ingestion of animal liver (in this case, the polar bear's) resulted in an excess of vitamin A which is toxic. It was not until Admiral Robert E. Peary's fourth and finally successful push to the North Pole in 1909 that he learned how to eat as an Eskimo eats and thereby avoided vitamin A toxicity.

OTHER ESSENTIAL MICRONUTRIENTS

There are compounds other than vitamins that must of necessity be in our diet for us to live healthy lives. Since these substances can be derived from other sources, they are not routinely accepted as vitamins. One such is choline, an essential ingredient in some fats (such as lecithin, found in egg yolk) and of acetylcholine, an important neurotransmitter. Choline can be synthesized from the amino acid, serine. The richest food sources are heart, brain, and egg yolks. Supplements, of course, are available. They have been found useful in some cases of Alzheimer-type memory loss problems.

Another essential micronutrient is inositol, which is an important component of myelin, the insulating sheath that protects nerves. In cases of peripheral neuropathy such as occurs in diabetes and Guillian-Barre disease, inositol supplements can be very useful. Also, as a phosphorylated compound, it functions as a "second messenger" for hormones intracellularly. Good dietary sources are muscle (especially shark muscle), heart, whole grains, beans, and nuts.

A third example is butyric acid, a short chain (4 carbon) unsaturated fatty acid found in small amounts in animal fats. This fat, rather than glucose, as customary in other cells of the body, is used as the energy source for the work done by our intestinal lining cells in absorbing nutrients from various foods. Without butyric acid (or butyrate), our digestion of vegetables is hindered and may be a cause of malabsorption syndrome. One of the best sources of butyric acid is butter, which may explain the prevailing custom of adding a bit of butter to the various vegetables we eat. Some butyric acid is also synthesized by bacteria in the gut.

It is extremely likely that, as research advances, other specific compounds will be found that fit this category of non-vitamin essential nutrients.

FIBER
Fiber refers to the indigestible residue of plants. They are complex carbohydrates made in such a way that we are unable to digest them. They encompass a wide variety of molecular structures that differ in their degree of solubility in water. They all, however, do have important health effects. In general, they add to the bulk of bowel con-

tents and stimulate the passage thereof. Shorter transit times (time of ingestion of food until its elimination via defecation) are related to decreased incidence of colon cancer. Water-soluble fiber tends to decrease cholesterol levels. A listing of common food fibers follows:

Water insoluble	Partially soluble	Water soluble
Wheat bran cereals	Kidney beans	Apples
Wheat products	Navy beans	Bananas
Brown rice	Green beans	Citrus
Cooked lentils	Green peas	Carrots
	Barley	
	Oats	

If one looks at the incidence of diseases among various populations around the world, a relationship to the intake of vegetable and grain fiber becomes apparent. The man who deserves the greatest credit for bringing this to the world's attention is Dr. Denis Burkitt of England. A summary of his observations on the importance of fiber follows:

> Until the past six or seven generations, man ate a diet filled with vegetables and grain fiber. With industrialization in "Westernized" populations, the diet changed greatly; the processing of foods for commercial sale and the selection of foods resulted in the loss of much of the fiber present in diet, especially of grain foods. Comparing the illnesses occurring in industrialized and non-industrialized populations, it is apparent that many of our more common illnesses simply do not occur, or occur very rarely, in the less industrialized areas. Such illnesses are diabetes, constipation, diverticulitis, colon cancer, heart disease and other atherosclerotic ills, obesity, gall bladder disease and gallstones, pancreatitis, hiatal hernia, appendicitis, hemorrhoids, varicose veins, and even breast cancer. The epidemiologic relationship of these diseases to the lack of adequate dietary fiber is unmistakable. We don't completely understand the physiological mechanisms that underlie this relationship, but the validity of the linkage is solid. The question is: how did this come about and what are we going to do about it?

In Northern climes, man's food through the winter months included, of necessity, those foods that could be stored, i.e., cereal grains, legumes, and tubers. Other vegetables and fruits were eaten only in summer seasons. The grains, legumes, and tubers provided a high fiber diet. Now we've thrown out those foods and substituted hamburgers, French fries, the cola drinks, fruit and salad vegetables that lack the fiber we need.

The benefits of fiber are many. Fiber adds bulk and retains water in our stools for easier, more prompt passage, thus reducing the development of hemorrhoids, varicose veins, and hiatal hernia. Fiber alters the bacteria in the intestine for better digestion and reduces the conversion of primary into secondary bile acids, which are potential cancer promoters; it absorbs more bile acids and dilutes them within a larger stool mass, thus protecting against colon cancer. With fiber, the bile itself is more soluble and less likely to form gall stones; similarly, fiber protects against pancreatitis by preventing biliary sludge. Fiber reduces one's fat absorption and lowers cholesterol levels, thus reducing coronary heart disease risk. The fiber in grains is especially healthful but, despite all the information printed on bread wrappers, it is difficult to find a supermarket bread still containing its full complement of fiber.

A good way to test your need for more fiber is the bowel transit time test. The bowel transit time is the time it takes for food to travel from ingestion to exit via the bowels. All that is needed is to eat some food that can serve as a marker when it appears in the stool. Fresh corn on the cob is one such food; we digest the starch within the kernels but not the kernels themselves, which will be visible in the bowel movement, when they are passed. Simply eat some corn and watch your bowel movements until you see the kernels. That is your bowel transit time. A healthy transit time is 18-24 hours. In the US, common bowel transit times are found to be 2-3 days. If such is found, it is an excellent sign you need more fiber and water in your diet.

It is difficult to imagine a more cost-effective way of reducing degenerative disease in our society than to return to a proper high fiber diet. I can think of no better example of the axiom that prevention is far better than treatment. In this case, prevention involves merely a return to a proper diet. If enough people demand these foods, our agriculture business will provide them.

ANTIOXIDANTS

"Free radicals" are single atoms or molecules with an unpaired electron in their outer electron ring. They are extremely chemically reactive. Free radicals are routinely created in body metabolism but also result from exposure to such diverse pollutants as radiation, smog, chlorine, certain food additives, benzene, or benzopyrene (cigarette smoke). Free radicals steal electrons from neighboring molecules, thus initiating a chain reaction among thousands of molecules, especially the fat molecules within cell membranes, causing the ruination of cells, damaged DNA, cell mutation leading to cancer, and arterial wall damage leading to plaque formation. Since singlet oxygen or oxygen radicals are often the chemical units carrying the electron charge, these chemical assaults are called oxidation reactions; our molecular defenders are called antioxidants. Among our antioxidant defenders, the most well-known are vitamin C, vitamin E, vitamin A, and the mineral selenium. Given the polluted nature of our environment, it is essential to keep our bodies well supplied with these nutrients.

Recent large studies have confirmed that antioxidants, and particularly vitamin E, are protective against heart deaths. These Harvard-based tests of large numbers of both men and women found, after correction for all other known factors, that heart deaths were approximately 60% lower in those taking vitamin E. It can be reliably expected that more and more disease states will be found to have an oxidation factor in their etiology and that the story of antioxidants is far from complete.

GRAIN: THE STAFF OF LIFE

Before leaving this fascinating topic of nutrition, it might be wise to review the wonder of grain, i.e., the seeds of plants. These small round kernels by which plants propagate are truly amazing. They fall to the ground, some float in the wind, and others survive the passage through the intestines of animals that eat them. Most grains can lie dormant through alternating seasons (even years) until a propitious time for germination. Their durability stems from their outer fibrous coat, which is laced with the water-soluble vitamins and proteins, and armored with minerals making them impervious to inclement conditions. The bulk of the seed is the endosperm, a load of carbohydrate starch that will provide the nutrition for the embryo plant when it germinates. Within the endosperm is the plant germ, the latent embryo of the plant-to-be, with its magic complement of the fat-soluble vitamins and high-energy unsaturated fatty acids upon which we have come to depend. When eaten whole and combined with a diet of protein sufficiency, humans benefit mightily from these amazing seeds, consuming them as cereals, pasta, or bread. Great civilizations arose where grain-growing was successful, the classic examples being the valleys of the Tigris and Euphrates rivers (the "Fertile Crescent") and of the Nile in Egypt.

The modern processing of foods, however, has been a disaster as far as grains are concerned. In the pursuit of a longer shelf life, our bakers use milled grain (removal of the protective outer fibrous coat along with its minerals, proteins, and water-soluble vitamins) and discarding the grain germ (the fats in them go rancid when exposed to air), leaving only the nutrient-deficient endosperm starch for the making of the bread, pasta, pastries, and cereals filling our supermarket shelves. These are the empty calories that have replaced the nutrient-rich grains of our predecessors. This the white fluffy starch sold to us with proud names such as "Gold Medal" flour which is best put to use by grade school pupils to make paste for gluing papers together. The milled-off grain fibers are sometimes sold back to us as bran. The loss of the grain germ is the chief reason for the prevalent deficiency in vitamin E. And the marketing gurus of food processors call this progress.

A word to the wise: buy only <u>whole grain</u> products. Do not be fooled by items labeled 100% this or that grain; such labels mean only that other grains were not included and do not mean that the whole grain was used in the food product so advertised.

SELF QUIZ

1. The chief source of our dietary minerals is
   _____ .

2. When vegetables are cooked in water, many of the minerals dissolve into the water and are lost. True or False?

3. Microwave cooking damages food-borne minerals. True or False?

4. Sodium intake comes mainly from the salt shaker. True or False?

5. Typical daily sodium intake is _____ mg/day and the typical daily requirement is _____ mg/day.

6. Sodium intake is toxic only when insufficiently balanced with potassium. True or False?

7. Where do cows get their calcium?
   _____

8. Name the fat-soluble vitamins. _____, _____, _____, and _____.

9. With adequate dietary fiber, healthy intestinal transit time is _____hrs.

10. Antioxidants protect us from "free radical" toxicity; can you name them? _____, _____, _____, _____.

Answers can be found on page 85.

CHAPTER SIX
STRESS

<u>PART ONE:</u> THE LIMBIC BRAIN
NEUROANATOMY

When one looks at a picture of the brain, one usually is presented with its outward appearance. If a cross section is presented, one can see gray matter and white matter. The gray matter contains brain cells and the white matter contains the neurons connecting one portion of the brain with another portion or with the spinal cord. The white matter is white because the neurons are covered with protective myelin insulation, the neurolemma. In the middle of the brain is a thick band of white matter (the corpus callosum) that contains the nerve fibers connecting one side of the brain with the other. Immediately below the corpus callosum and surrounding the lateral ventricles lies another mass of gray matter (the limbic brain) below which is nestled the pituitary gland.

The big top brain serves our consciousness and our primary senses such as sight, sound, touch, sense of location, etc. It contains our speech center and allows us to be introspective, cogitate in abstractions, and fret about the future. The smaller, more ancient brain lying beneath the corpus callosum serves a different master beyond our force of will - it is the limbic brain which is the center for homeostasis, and the sensation and the expression of our emotions. It contains areas of the brain we call the hippocampus (vital to memory and unconscious learning), the thalamus, the hypothalamus and the mammillary bodies and many other centers, some of which we have not yet named but they all act as permanently running computers to keep track of all our bodily functions. These centers formulate the messages (endorphins) that tell the pituitary what messages (the trophic hormones) to send to our endocrine systems. Endorphin receptor sites, once thought to be confined to the brain and central nervous system, have now been found throughout the body, including heart muscle, the stomach, and even in the joints of our skeleton. The body and mind are one.

FUNCTION OF THE LIMBIC BRAIN

We all probably know that the expressions for grief, anger, delight, laughter, and fear are universal among humans and that they are not learned but are innate. Even a baby at 24 hours will respond to facial expressions of these emotions with identical expressions of his own. How does the baby know how to do that? The answer is that these reactions are built into the limbic brain. Music that stirs a martial fervor, that is calming, that is dissonant or sad is felt the same way by all, despite great differences in cultural settings. That, too, is built into the limbic brain.

Have you ever wondered how the body knows when and how much to sweat, how it increases its heart output to compensate for change in demand, what controls thyroid production, insulin secretion, urine output, etc.? How does the body know when to increase its white blood cell count? And where is the thermostat that controls our stable body temperature? These and more are all in the limbic brain. If we had to keep track of all our autonomic functions consciously, we wouldn't have the brain power to know our own name. The body does that for us and the center for all these computers is the limbic brain.

THE FOUR "Fs"

The majority of the functions of the limbic brain can be said to be pre-programmed, i.e., genetically set and not a result of being learned. The scope of the programs is awesome, affecting everything from basic autonomic nerve system function (sympathetic and parasympathetic) to subtle variations in personality characteristics. The neural centers controlling this vast array of responses are interrelated in a way typical of analog computers, operating as software programs integrated with the hard disk of the neural chassis to create the broad spectrum of ever-varying physiologic fluctuations of our neuro-immuno-hormonal regulatory system. The individual response patterns are referred to as "drives" and the more important ones are called "primary drives." The teleologic focus of the entire system is preservation of the species, if not the self. As members of the human species, we are driven to seek food and water, to fight to defend our lives, to flee from truly dangerous circumstances, and to procreate. A favorite mnemonic, undoubtedly coined by some waggish medical student, to aid in remembering these four primary drives is the four Fs which are Feeding, Fight, Flight, and Sex.

RELATION TO OPTIMAL HEALTH

Within the limbic brain are sensors for hormone levels. If one or another is too high or too low, polypeptide signals (endorphins) are sent via special tiny veins to the pituitary gland which, in response, sends its own trophic hormones through the blood stream to tell the specific endocrine gland to speed up or slow down the production of the hormone in question. This is an ongoing process in maintaining optimal health.

These sensors are sensitive to events going on all over the body at all times. Some events excite the sensor and some can depress it. No action or reaction of any part of the body is independent in and of itself. It is not unlike a symphony orchestra, but immensely larger and more complex. If the trumpet section is playing too fast, it may throw off the cellos sitting nearby. If there is not sufficient rosin on the violinists' bows, their strings will squeal and the audience (i.e., body) will stir uncomfortably. Experiments show that a mild electric current to an anterior portion of the hypothalamus will cause a shower of hydrochloric acid in the stomach; the same electric current applied to the posterior portion of the hypothalamus will send the victim into a deep, suicidal depression.

Sometimes the demands on the computers of the limbic brain are contradictory or confusing to its programs or simply excessive for its capability. Let us look at one such example.

"HYPOGLYCEMIA"

In the ventromedial nucleus of the hypothalamus in the limbic brain is a small cluster of brain cells that serves as the body's glucose regulator, or glucostat. When sugar passes over our tongue, we sense (via cranial nerve IX) a sweet taste and, thereby, input of sugar is detected by this glucostat. As we know, sugar requires little digestion, and absorption is rapid. The sudden surge of sugar must be met by a surge of insulin for it to be used by muscle cells or brain cells or simply stored in fat cells for conversion to fat. This is the job of the glucostat, to estimate the sugar intake and regulate the secretion of pancreatic release of insulin. By evolution, the computer is designed to handle only modest amounts of sugar at any one time because that is the nature of unprocessed food. Now, however, the demands on the glucostat are different. A can of regular Coca Cola provides 9 teaspoons of sugar. One would have to eat over 30 feet of sugar cane to get that much sugar. Crystallized sugar was invented only a century or two ago. A milkshake might provide a quarter pound of sugar. Sugar surges of this magnitude may exceed the capacity of a person's glucostat. Its signal to the pancreas may be in error; too much insulin may be released into the blood stream.

When excessive insulin floods into the blood stream, it causes the transfer into cells of not only all the sugar that was eaten but also a good portion of the sugar that was already there for general purposes. Blood sugar level falls. If it falls too far or too fast, the computer switches gears and sends a signal to the adrenal glands to secrete adrenalin which has the effect of releasing stored sugar (i.e., glycogen) from the liver into the blood stream to bring the blood sugar back to normal. This solves the blood sugar problem but now the body has all this adrenalin to deal with. Adrenalin (fight or flight hormone) is our response to sudden stress, as would happen in an automobile accident or an earthquake or being slapped on the face. It causes our pupils to dilate, our heart races, our blood pressure rises, our muscles tense, our stomach tightens and we experience a rising sense of anxiety.

When all this happens without apparent provocation, our thinking rationalizing brain sometimes concocts a provocative scenario; the radio's too loud, someone's comment on the president's competence is offensive, or our child's behavior is insulting. Our reaction is disproportionate to the assumed offense but we fail to "see" it because the reaction to the adrenalin surge is so real.

Now imagine all this happening when the limbic brain is coping with stresses from other sources as well. In fact, the abnormal glucostat action may only happen when other sources of stress have, in effect, turned up its voltage. It may only happen when the background blood sugar is already running a bit low. It may only happen when a certain amount of alcohol is also on board or at certain times of the day when our adrenal steroids (which also have a say in blood sugar levels) are in low supply.

I think you can see the complexity and the frustration that stems from an illness such as reactive hypoglycemia, described above. Linear thinkers will have particular difficulty with it. And this is only the tip of the iceberg. From this and other limbic computers can come dysfunctional and conflicting messages to all parts of the body and to all aspects of our mental and emotional outlook. Within the limbic brain are central controls for our digestive system, blood pressure, vascular tone (cold, sweaty feet), immune system (a positive outlook may protect us from infections), muscle tone (headaches, backaches), sexual urges, sleep patterns, thyroid and other endocrine gland function, and many, many other body systems. What a shame that medical schools teach so little about this important brain center.

FURTHER CONSIDERATIONS: For most of us, willful or voluntary control over any limbic brain function is generally beyond us. Some yogis develop some control, at least temporarily, over some of these functions. Transcendental meditation may do something of the same. So might hypnosis, directed suggestions, acupuncture, and the ever-widening circle of "alternative" therapies that have arisen. The body has vast powers of healing, most of which we probably never utilize. There is much to be learned about the limbic brain and much to be gained by doing so; it is time we got on with it.

PART TWO: THE STRESS OF LIFE

In 1955, when I was finishing medical school in Minnesota, Hans Selye was in Montreal finishing his classic book defining stress, *The Stress of Life*. I encourage anyone interested in understanding stress to read it. In it, he extended the definition of stress from the previous concept of "the rate of wear and tear in the body" to the General Adaptation Syndrome which develops in three stages: (1) the alarm reaction; (2) the stage of resistance; and (3) the stage of exhaustion. He did not "discover" stress; he was the first to assign a word to the general idea of wear and tear that all creatures experience, define it in an objective manner, and live long enough to see it become understood and accepted around the world. Many languages did not have a word carrying this meaning of stress.

To understand stress, it is necessary to understand the concept of *homeostasis* as taught by Claude Bernard in Paris in the 1860s. Though he did not use that specific word, he taught that one of the most characteristic features of all living things is their ability to maintain the constancy of their internal milieu despite changes in their surroundings. Walter B. Cannon, a famous Harvard physiologist, subsequently (early 1900s), called this power to maintain internal constancy "homeostasis." One's body tries to keep its internal temperature a constant 98.6° F, its water intake in balance with water loss, its blood flow and pressure within proper limits, its serum levels of nutrients, minerals, and acidity within precise limits, its number of red blood cells in proper limits, etc., etc. As we saw in the case of hypoglycemia, there are automatic mechanisms to keep blood glucose levels stable. The same is true within each cell of the body. To live is to strive to maintain a relatively constant internal environment.

Working against this are all the fluctuations in our surroundings; changes in temperature, lack of water, irregular feedings, the presence of toxins, assaults by virulent germs, trauma to body tissues, lack of rest, periodic gluts of unneeded fats or deficiencies of essential nutrients, etc. The destabilizing agents need not be physical; we may experience conflicting emotional drives or needs which, via the limbic brain, disrupt the harmony of the body's physiologic responses.

Twenty-four centuries ago, Hippocrates taught his students that disease consists of two elements: "pathos" (suffering) and "ponos" (the fight of the body to restore itself toward normal). Disease is not the surrender of the body to illness; disease is also the fight for health. This fight, this toil, this striving of the body to restore the normal state is what we now call Stress.

The agents that induce the destabilization from normal are called the Stressors. The manifestations that occur in the body during times of stress are called the Stress Reaction. Stress, itself, is the common denominator of all the adaptive reactions by the body. It is not the set of reactions, nor is it the specific agents that trigger the reactions. Stress is the struggle to regain homeostasis. Stress is the state manifested by the set of nonspecific changes induced by "ponos," regardless of cause.

In Dr. Selye's depiction of stress mechanism relationships, stressors affect the brain to cause (1) trophic hormone messages to the thyroid gland, adrenals, gonads, and muscles, and (2) direct neural stimulation of adrenaline and acetylcholine.

These, in turn, affect changes in thyroid hormone, adrenalin, liver function, cortisol, heart, blood vessels, kidney function, muscle tension, white blood cells and other immune system function, sweat glands, and thymus function. Further, all these affects are also modulated by conditioning responses. That is, stressor effect may be up- or down-regulated by prior experiences or other confounding conditions.

Dr. Selye's list of diseases resulting from stress included the following:	
Hypertension	Emotional illness
Heart disease	Diabetes
Kidney disease	Cancer
Rheumatoid arthritis	Headache
Gastrointestinal disease	Backache
Allergies	Tendonitis, bursitis
Autoimmune disorders	

We now know that the actual list of stress-induced diseases is much more extensive than the above.

Lessons to be learned, according to Dr. Selye, are:

1. that our body can meet the most diverse aggressions with the same adaptive defensive mechanism, and

2. that it is possible to dissect this mechanism so as to identify its ingredients objectively, and

3. that we need this kind of information to lay the scientific foundations for a new type of treatment, whose essence is to combat disease by strengthening the body's own defenses against stress.

Is stress bad? No, stress is an inherent adaptive mechanism by which we restore homeostasis and create healing and gain strengths. It is only when these mechanisms become exhausted or misdirected by unusual conditioning or genetic error that stress can lead to bad results.

What about emotional stress? Here I find it useful to think in terms of conflicting primary drives. Primary drives are those undeniable emotional and behavioral response patterns triggered by conditions to which we are innately predisposed and which evoke pleasure or discomfort, such as feeding or sexual drives. But these also include colors, musical sounds, the sense of proportion in spatial objects, assertiveness or compliance, tendencies of being outgoing or shy, daring or cautious, etc. Primary drives also refer to modes of thinking such as a preference for tactile versus abstract, etc.

When a conflict of primary drives occurs, it may not connote a conflict of "good" versus "bad," but more often is a conflict between two "good" drives. For example, a young man may have a strong drive to be a good son and follow the wishes of his parents, while at the same time he may be influenced by peer pressure or merely have a strong drive to be on his own and seek his own fortune in the world, a path that may conflict with his parents' wishes. This often happens in one's college years and he may go through a difficult period of resolution of this conflict in drives. We may have a need to be loved by our children, yet we also recognize the need to discipline them and risk that love. These are, of course, quite normal conflicts. Surprisingly, they can create stress of such strength that physiologic responses do occur affecting, perhaps, sleep, digestion, muscle tension, etc.

The deeper and stronger the nature of the conflicting drives, the more difficult is the resolution of the conflict and the greater the physiologic responses. The longer the lack of resolution persists, the more likely is the development of a disease ("dis-ease"). If merely the symptoms are treated (e.g., tranquilizers, antidepressants), a paradox ensues: the more successful the treatment is, the less likely it is that the deeper conflict of primary drives will be resolved.

Some unresolved conflicts can be tolerated (usually as chronic anxiety symptoms) for a long time. If they are deep and strong, however, the lack of resolution can lead to exhaustion of our adaptation mechanisms, leading to depression. Depression involves a loss in our will to cope and makes spontaneous recovery much less likely.

It is apparent that sometimes we need help in resolving conflicts of primary drives (mental stress). It is here that we can learn techniques for coping, seek out the insights gained from psychology, spiritual counselors, and others who have gone before, strive to be open to the healing influences of friendship, sharing, music, the arts, and come to terms with life's limitations and, also, its glories. No one is immune to stress, no life is free of it, and no single path will do for all individuals or their conditions. Humans have the gift of self-consciousness, introspection, and the contemplation of the future. It is also our burden. We are all seekers of the art of coping.

SELF QUIZ

1. Mental attitude has an effect on bodily functions. True or False?

2. Getting heartburn when upset is an example of (a) a stressor, (b) stress, or (c) a stress reaction. Pick one.

3. The pituitary, in releasing its trophic hormones to other glands, does so in response to endorphin signals from limbic brain sensors. True or False?

4. The limbic brain is the center of our autonomic nervous system. True or False?

5. Stress is generally bad for us. True or False?

6. Sugar can induce dysfunctional responses in some people. True or False?

7. Learning is a function of (a) cerebral cortex, (b) limbic cortex or (c) both. Pick one.

8. One's emotions can affect one's cholesterol level. True or False?

9. Brain function and body function should be considered separate entities. True or False?

10. I.Q. (intelligence quotient) is unrelated to nutrition. True or False?

Answers are on the page 85.

CHAPTER SEVEN
FUNDAMENTALS OF EXERCISE

We are animals that thrive on exercise, are meant to exercise, and many of us living in the US today manage to live a life almost devoid of exercise. The results are not good. Muscle disuse leads to the following:

— our muscle cells lose the enzyme capacity to maintain energy

— our tendons and ligaments lose their strength and flexibility (a common injury is the ruptured Achilles tendon that occurs when a sedentary 50-year-old decides to take up tennis)

— our cells accumulate lactic acid with even mild exertion and we suffer aches and pains

— the caliber of our arteries decreases

— our food is converted to fats rather than used for energy

— we make less noradrenalin and are subject to depression

— our ability to provide our body with oxygen decays

— our muscles (including our heart) become flabby

— our bones become porous and more fragile

In sum, we tire more easily, hurt more, and fall apart more readily. Why do we do this to ourselves?

There are as many different ways to exercise as there are songs to sing. Exercise need not be onerous nor must we aspire to be star athletes. All the body wants is a little workout each day, a little sweat on the brow, a little fresh air in our lungs. Let us look at a few body mechanisms that benefit from exercise.

(1) Our primary cellular fuel is glucose... a simple molecule loaded with oxygen. Yet, even it requires additional oxygen prior to the energy payoff. Unless we exercise, our appropriate intracellular enzymes diminish and allow lactic acid accumulation, which leads to muscle cramps. Fat is also a wonderful fuel for our muscle cells but it requires even more oxygen than glucose. Its metabolism in the energy pathway is even less likely to be completed if we are not fit. When we are fit, by reason of exercise, we easily burn dietary fat for energy fuel. When we are not fit, the fat ends up in storage. When we are fit, we burn sugar for energy even when we are sitting down. Exercise is the key.

(2) Exercise, in burning off calories for energy, prevents their conversion into fat. This same process can lower one's cholesterol levels and, at the same time, will result in less LDL cholesterol and more HDL cholesterol, which is an added benefit.

(3) It has also been shown that exercise, in utilizing dietary sugars for energy, significantly decreases one's likelihood of developing non-insulin dependent diabetes mellitus (NIDDM).

(4) Muscle is composed of bundles containing many small muscle fibers. In any given action, a muscle will use only enough fibers to perform the action. By increasing a muscle workout, more muscle fibers are stimulated to respond, and more enzymes are created to convert stored energy (i.e., muscle glycogen) into work energy. This is called improved muscle tone. Heavyweight lifting is not necessary for this. With heavy lifting workouts ("pumping iron"), muscle cells will greatly increase muscle glycogen content, creating bigger muscles. (This muscle build-up, of itself, is not necessarily a health benefit.)

(5) When we exercise, our heart muscle is strengthened and our arteries increase in caliber. Larger arteries not only carry more blood better but they can tolerate a given burden of cholesterol deposits with less danger of obstruction. Also, our lungs become better at

absorbing oxygen from air and transporting it to the blood stream. It is even good for menopausal hot flashes.

(6) Many of our bodies' aches and pains are from muscle imbalance - our flexors overpower our extenders and we hunch over in a posture that is bad for our backs, necks, shoulders, and arms. We lose flexibility as well as strength. A few minutes of exercise each morning is frequently all that we need.

(7) Bones not put to the stress of exercise lose bone mass and are more likely to fracture. This lack of exercise is probably the greatest cause of the osteoporosis epidemic presently upon us.

(8) As most of us know, exercise is excellent for correcting constipation.

Need one say more?

Despite the small size of this chapter, the exercise factor is just as important as any of the others. I will leave it to the ingenuity and individuality of the reader to find his or her best and most enjoyable exercises.

SELF QUIZ

1. Relatively light exercise will increase muscle tone. True or False?

2. Heavy exercise builds big muscles; this makes us healthier. True or False?

3. Exercise is good for muscles but has no effect on bones. True or False?

4. Exercise can improve one's total cholesterol/HDL cholesterol ratio. True or False?

5. Exercise, to be beneficial, must be performed to the point of discomfort. True or False?

6. The physical fitness of US schoolchildren, compared to a generation ago, is (1) better, (b) the same, or (c) worse. Pick one.

7. Exercise which improves the cellular oxygen supply is called (a) aerobic, or (b) anaerobic. Pick one.

8. Aerobic exercise is good for hot flashes in women. True or False?

9. A weight loss program using diet alone is just as healthy for you as a weight loss program that includes exercise. True or False?

10. Exercise in the morning can increase energy throughout the whole day. True or False?

Answers can be found on page 85.

CHAPTER EIGHT
SUMMARY

The concepts and fundamentals of optimal health discussed above have included a description of (1) nutrition, in particular the role of carbohydrates, fats, proteins, vitamins, minerals, and fiber; (2) an understanding of what is meant by stress; and (3) some idea of the importance of exercise. We have seen that excessive sugar intake (common in the standard American diet) is not good and that complex carbohydrates are better for us than refined carbohydrates. We have learned the complex role of fat and that the cholesterol story is a bit different than as commonly presented. We discovered, probably with some surprise, that excessive protein can be harmful to us. Hopefully, we have gained an modest appreciation of enzymes and the roles of vitamins and minerals. The concept of stress was presented in considerable detail with emphasis on its causes and its metabolic consequences. And, lastly, we surveyed the importance of exercise.

With these fundamentals in mind, put to yourself the following questions:

1. What is a salubrious environment?

2. What is meant by proper exercise?

3. How is stress to be managed?

4. Can anything be done about genetics?

5. What is a proper diet?

One of the keys in making progress with any problem is to ask the right questions. This is more important than memorizing answers. With the right questions and a basis of understanding the facts, the answers will come.

In regard to question #5, it may be helpful to consider the following:

Contrary to popular argument, there is but one diet beneficial to all the major health risks such as cardiovascular disease, osteoporosis, cancer, obesity, constipation, aging, and many degenerative diseases. Even one's resistance to infectious diseases has important nutritional and stress-related factors. The best diet emphasizes whole grains, legumes, and other vegetables, fruit, seafoods, allows eggs and olive oil, limits protein intake, and includes supplements of antioxidants such as vitamins C and E. Red meat should be used only in modest amounts, if at all. Homogenized milk should probably not be drunk by adults. Sugar and highly refined starches should be severely restricted. The diet should avoid processed foods and known toxins such as artificial coloring agents, fluoride, insecticides and herbicides to the greatest extent possible.

In the past, nutrition education has followed the Four Food Groups, so favored by the dairy and meat industry. With new understanding, a new and better food plan is emerging. Dairy and meat are demoted, as are sugar and refined starches. Vegetables are seen to be the major ingredients of a healthy diet.

The Old Diet	The New Diet
Meat	Legumes
Dairy	Vegetables
Grains	Whole grains
Fruit/vegetables	Fruit (with only minor use of sugar, refined starches,
(Discard this diet)	dairy & meat)

In the old standard American diet (SAD), 25% of the calorie intake was provided by sugar and often over 40% of the calories came from fat. This is nutritional nonsense. Protein provided 15% of the calories, leaving only 20% of one's calories to be derived from complex carbohydrates (legumes and vegetables)

The goal of the new diet is to limit sugar to 5% of the total calories and drastically reduce the use of feed lot meat and dairy fats. Whole grains, legumes and vegetables should provide 75-80% of our caloric intake. For those new to this way of thinking, the following partial lists of foods in these categories should be of help:

<u>Grains</u>	whole grain bread, cereal, corn, rice, millet, bulgur, buckwheat, and groats.
<u>Vegetables</u>	carrots, winter squash, sweet potatoes, pumpkin, broccoli, collards, kale, mustard and turnip greens, chicory, and bok choy.
<u>Legumes</u>	beans, peas, lentils, chickpeas, fermented soy products (tofu and tempeh).
<u>Fruit</u>	citrus fruit, melons, strawberries, and many others. Be sure to choose fresh whole fruit over fruit juices.

A good book for more information on the new four food group eating plan is *The Power of Your Plate* by Neal D. Barnard, MD, available from the Physicians Committee.

Typical diet composition in % of total calories.

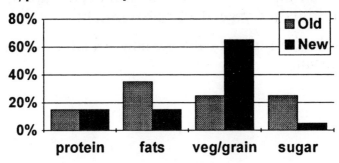

Most contemporary physicians will tell you that you can obtain all your vitamins and minerals from a good, well-balanced diet. This may have been true in Eden but it is not true in today's world of processed foods. The question of whether vitamin/mineral supplements are beneficial when taken in addition to a good, well-balanced diet was addressed in a report by Chandra RJ et al, "Effect of vitamin and trace-element supplementation on immune responses and infection in elderly subjects," *Lancet* 1992, vol. 340, 1124-27. A group of elderly individuals, average age 75, with good diets were randomly assigned to receive either placebo or a modest vitamin/mineral supplement daily for 12 months. In this blinded study, nutrient status and immunological variables were assessed at baseline and 12 months, and the frequency of illness due to infection was ascertained. Results indicated a "significant improvement of immunocompetence" and 40% fewer episodes of infection-related illnesses over the 12 months in the supplemented group. The authors conclude that "such an intervention led to striking reduction in illness, a finding that is of considerable clinical and public-health importance." Need one say more?

Remember that vitamins and minerals are just one part of an extensive complex balance of many other health factors. Note that in the reference above, the vitamin/mineral supplements were added to an otherwise well-balanced diet. Studies that isolate a single nutrient without regard to the whole spectrum of nutritional factors will usually fail to show benefit. The addition of any specific supplemental nutrient will do you little good if you lack the basic nutrients found in fresh, unprocessed plant foods. Your grandmother told you to eat your fruits and vegetables. She was right.

The basics of optimal health are now available to everyone. The rest is up to you.

ANSWERS TO SELF QUIZ QUESTIONS

Chapter 1.　The answer to all ten questions is False.

Chapter 2.　The answer to all ten questions is True.

Chapter 3.　1. true, 2. false, 3. false, 4. false, 5. true, 6. true, 7. true, 8. false, 9. HDL, LDL, 10. true

Chapter 4.　1. true, 2. true, 3. false, 4. true, 5. true, 6. false, 7. false, 8. nitrogen, 9. false, 10. true

Chapter 5.　1. plants, 2. true, 3. false, 4. false, 5. 8-10,000; 1500, 6. true, 7. From plants they eat, 8. vitamins A, D, E, and K, 9. 18-24 hrs, 10. vitamins C, E, A, and the mineral selenium.

Chapter 6.　1. true, 2. (c), 3. true, 4. true, 5. false, 6. true, 7. (c), 8. true, 9. false, 10. false.

Chapter 7.　1. true, 2. false, 3. false, 4. true, 5. false, 6. (c), 7. (a), 8. true, 9. false, 10. true

In the next section, Optimal Health Applications, the study of optimal health will apply these concepts and fundamentals to the prevention and amelioration of specific major illnesses. These illnesses will include heart disease, arteriosclerosis, hypertension and stroke, cancer, osteoporosis, the "degenerative" diseases, gastrointestinal diseases, and iatrogenic disease. The knowledge that exists today can substantially reduce our risks of these illnesses and enhance our pursuit of optimal health.

OPTIMAL HEALTH:

APPLICATIONS

Optimal health concepts and fundamentals will be applied to understanding the causes and prevention of the most common health issues in our society today.

Chapter 9. Cardiovascular disease, the number 1 killer in the United States, is largely a matter of atherosclerosis. This chapter will cover coronary heart disease, the role of diet and cholesterol, stress and exercise.

Chapter 10. Hypertension and Stroke: we learn about arteriosclerosis and what we can do to prevent it. We will review dietary factors, exercise, stress, environmental agents and learn strategies to protect our vascular system.

Chapter 11. Cancer: what can be done to prevent it and what can be done if we have it? The American Cancer Society admits that over 35% of cancers are nutrition-related. Nutritional and other environmental factors will be discussed.

Chapter 12. Osteoporosis: the most debilitating and expensive disease of women in the US. Learn the role of diet, exercise, and the gonadal hormones. A simple program for preventing and reversing osteoporosis will be presented.

Chapter 13. Degenerative diseases: are they simply the consequence of aging or are they due to factors of life style? This chapter will discuss arthritis, senility, Alzheimer's disease and other illnesses common in older life.

Chapter 14. Hyperacidity, peptic ulcer, and other gastrointestinal disorders: what are the new facts about diet and digestion? What about milk, meat, or fiber? What should we be eating these days to keep our G-I tract happy?

Chapter 15. Chronic fatigue syndrome and other frustrating 20th century illnesses. Conventional medical care is failing. What causes these "incurable" illnesses and what should be done?

Chapter 16. Iatrogenic disease: how to protect yourself when dealing with your doctor and still be a good patient. Over 25% of hospital admissions stem directly from mismanaged medications. Learn how to ask the right questions and demand responsible answers. It's your life, after all.

CARDIOVASCULAR DISEASE

Cardiovascular disease is the #1 degenerative disease of man-kind. In the US it is the underlying cause of 734,000 deaths a year. We are as old as our arteries are. Without a good heart and open arteries, no tissue can remain healthy or function normally. The enemy of our cardiovascular system is atherosclerosis, i.e., a thickening of the interior linings of our arteries that can lead to obstruction of blood flow. We see the results as exertional fatigue, claudication, angina and other heart problems, and strokes. If we can learn how our arteries got that way, we can then learn how to prevent it.

MECHANISM OF DEVELOPING ATHEROSCLEROSIS

Arteries are tubes carrying blood from the heart out to the tissues of the body. Some are as large as a garden hose (the aorta), some as small as a string, and the terminals (capillaries) are so small that red blood cells must travel through them one at a time. Arterial walls are constructed of three layers. The outer layer (adventitia) is tough and elastic; the middle layer (media) is composed of muscle cells that provide the ability for the artery to contract or dilate; the inner layer (intima) is composed of thin, plate-like, very smooth cells (endothelium). The smoothness is very important because blood contains platelets, which are designed to trigger clotting if they tumble over rough surfaces such as the edge of a torn artery. Within the arterial wall are extremely minute blood vessels (vaso vasorum) to bring nutrients and oxygen to the constituent cells.

Sometimes we absorb toxic agents into our blood stream, e.g., carbon monoxide and aromatic hydrocarbons from cigarette smoke. These highly reactive compounds can damage the endothelial cells or the underlying muscle cells of the middle arterial layer. This can result in a proliferation of muscle cells within this layer, a proliferation that exceeds the nutrient supply from the vaso vasorum and leads to cell death (necrosis) and degeneration of small areas. Cholesterol accumulates in these areas forming a mass that pushes up against the endothelial lining. An erosion of lining cells occurs and the cholesterol mass pushes out of the middle layer through this opening into the blood stream which carries it farther along until it finally clogs some arterial tributary downstream.

The same toxic agents will oxidize some cholesterol molecules, converting them to compounds that are more prone to become sticky and form plaques on the inner lining of our arteries. LDL-cholesterol is especially prone to oxidation, whereas HDL-cholesterol is relatively resistant. Trans-fatty acids increase LDL-cholesterol, whereas natural cis-fatty acids favor HDL-cholesterol. (See chapter 3.)

Platelets tend to aggregate at these areas and trap LDL-cholesterol in a matrix of platelets, fibrin, and cholesterol, thus contributing to the plaque formation on the inside of the artery. Being an irregularity of the general smoothness of the endothelium, they gradually grow as they acquire more platelets and more cholesterol and eventually cause a significant narrowing of the artery lumen. HDL-cholesterol does not stick to artery walls as LDL-cholesterol does.

The coronary arteries (those that sit on the surface of the heart and bring blood to the heart muscle) are particularly prone to this type of damage because they are constantly bending and stretching with each heart beat. The cholesterol that gathers within these arteries is similar to a soft wax. In angioplasty, these cholesterol collections can actually be pushed aside to make the artery opening (lumen) bigger or, with a laser, they can be vaporized into carbon dioxide and water. Unfortunately, the endothelial lining cells are somewhat damaged in the procedure and cholesterol plaques start all over again, a process called restenosis, which then leads to open-heart coronary artery surgery.

The same process, of course, occurs elsewhere throughout the vascular system, e.g., groin, leg, neck and head arteries. When leg arteries become narrowed, exertion such as walking can cause leg cramps and pains that subside with rest. This is called *claudication*. In the neck, the carotid arteries carry blood to the head and brain. If plaques build up in these, fragments may break off and be carried with the blood to smaller arteries in the brain where they obstruct blood flow, thus depriving some brain cells of their needed oxygen and nutrients. This is called a *thrombo-embolic* stroke. If it involves only a tiny artery, the damage is not severe and the brain cells can recover because of nutrient arteries from nearby areas. If brief and involving no residual damage, this is called a *transient ischemic attack* or TIA . With high blood pressure, some strokes are caused by a rupture of an artery in the brain causing hemorrhage and, usually, a greater amount of initial damage. These can, however, heal and the area of damage will reduce considerably.

PREVENTION OF ATHEROSCLEROSIS

As is apparent, prevention is far better than treatment. Here again, the best prevention is a proper diet and avoidance of toxic oxidants. Foods that promote atherosclerosis are called *atherogenic*. By overindulgence, sugars, starches, and most fats all become atherogenic. As mentioned above, trans-fatty acids are more atherogenic than natural, or cis-fatty acids. In addition, one's individual atherogenic tendency has a genetic component not necessarily related to obesity. That is, many overweight people have no more atherosclerosis than slim or medium-weight people do. Any person with a family history of atherosclerosis would be wise, however, to avoid becoming overweight. The importance of weight has to do with how it is distributed. A good marker for atherosclerotic risk is the ratio between one's girth and one's height. The larger the girth/height ratio, the greater the risk.

Persons with diabetes are at special risk since diabetes connotes a defect in energy metabolism for both sugar and fat. Their LDL-cholesterol levels are higher, and their arteries develop a thickening of their walls unrelated to serum cholesterol. In middle age, their risk of having a heart attack is 12 times that of a non-diabetic. Diet and exercise, especially in early life, are very important.

If sugars and refined starches (pastries, etc.) can be kept to a minimum, one can then focus on fats. Certain fats are not atherogenic and should be encouraged; others are so-so; and a special group is definitely dangerous. The "good" fats are found in fish, olive and flaxseed oil, fresh vegetables, seeds and nuts, and shell fish. "Neutral" fats would be eggs and free range animals. The "bad" fats are processed oils, dairy fats, margarine, most "feed lot" red meats, pressed grain or nut oils, and any hydrogenated oil. A good book concerning this subject is *Fats that Heal, Fats that Kill* by Udo Erasmus, available as a paperback.

In addition to diet, exercise during one's early years is helpful. Exercise tends to increase the caliber of one's arteries. Thus, if atherosclerosis develops later in life, the size of the arterial lumen allows the presence of the developing plaques without becoming obstructed. Exercise also consumes extra calories and leaves less sugars and fats to be turned into cholesterol. Once the exercise stops, atherosclerosis resumes and diet becomes paramount again. Thus the cardiovascular fate of professional athletes is often worse than in the non-athlete if they continue their rich diet after their competitive years.

Women, on the other hand, are protected against atherosclerosis during their reproductive years. It is only after menopause that their risk begins to mirror the male pattern. This suggests that the female hormones probably have something to do with this protection. Estrogen, given to men, does not protect them, however, but actually increases their atherogenic risk. Estrogen (as estradiol-17ß), however, is a vasoactive hormone, causing relaxation of coronary arteries and increased blood flow in peripheral vascular beds and thus may have a beneficial effect on myocardial ischemia and lowered peripheral vascular resistance in women. Progesterone improves cellular oxygen utilization and decreases the formation and accumulation of cholesterol within the coronary arteries. The two female hormones together are probably more protective than estrogen alone. Hormone supplementation using low-dose estrogen and progesterone after menopause does not increase a woman's risk of atherosclerosis and may, in fact, prevent it. Estrogen plus syn-thetic progestins, however, lack this benefit and have been found to increase the risk of coronary artery spasm. (See below.)

Further, it has been suggested that monthly menstruation may be beneficial in this regard. A lower body load of iron may provide atherogenic protection.

CORONARY ARTERY DISEASE

The major cause of heart disease these days is a disease of the coronary arteries. This has not always been so. In 1916, Paul Dudley White, our first US cardiologist, performed an autopsy study of 1000 males who had died of heart disease. He found that younger males had died of rheumatic heart disease (later found to be due to child-hood streptococcus infections) and congenital heart defects; older males died of syphilitic disease of the aortic valve and tuberculosis heart problems. There were very few middle aged men who died of heart disease. Fifty years later, the same doctor did the same study and found an entirely different picture. Rheumatic heart trouble was very rare (penicillin kills streptococcus) and congenital heart abnormalities were being corrected by skillful surgery. Both tuberculosis and syphilis had become rare. Most of the men who had died of heart disease were middle aged (35-55) and essentially all had a new disease, i.e., block-age within the coronary arteries.

Coronary arteries are different in certain ways from other arter-ies throughout the body. They lie on the surface of a pulsating muscle mass, twisting and stretching with every beat; they nourish a muscle that never rests as other muscles do; they lack collateral branches that connect with other arteries; and they are more exposed (not being embedded in the muscle they serve) to damage by micro-waves, X-rays, and other radiation.

The disease Dr. White found in 1966 could not have been missed in his study of 50 years earlier: these arteries he examined in the '60s were obviously clogged with fatty material, i.e., cholesterol. The disease these men died of is called coronary heart disease (CHD) or coronary artery disease (CAD).

THE CHOLESTEROL THEORY OF CHD

Something had happened between 1916 and 1966 to cause this apparently new disease. Where had all this cholesterol clogging come from? Research begun in the '50s had focused on cholesterol. Dr. Ancel Keyes, a pharmacologist, discovered that, in the selection of countries he investigated, CHD correlated with elevated serum cholesterol. His research did *not* show that eating more cholesterol either raised serum cholesterol levels or was correlated with increased risk of CHD.

Nevertheless, the assumption was made (and exists today) that cholesterol in the diet was the source of cholesterol in blood that became the cholesterol lining these arteries and choking the blood flow to the heart muscle. Only later was it discovered (remembered) that we, as other animals do, synthesize our own cholesterol. Now the question becomes: if it is not the cholesterol we eat, what does cause us to make too much cholesterol?

Dr. White felt it was a combination of two or three factors: (1) something in the diet (probably the fats) that increased or altered our cholesterol; (2) a decrease in exercise as a consequence of changes in transportation and job characteristics made us more susceptible to this problem; and (3) probably stress. Dr. White recommended a return to eating fresh, unprocessed foods and a increase in exercise for which he, himself, took to riding a bicycle for the rest of his life. He also advocated a more relaxed, more humorous approach to life in general.

The question of the dietary elements is still widely debated. The idea of cholesterol in the diet causing the cholesterol in our arteries, though wrong, is neat and quite attractive. The problem is that reducing dietary cholesterol does *not* significantly reduce one's blood cholesterol or risk of heart disease. Also, other populations with high cholesterol intake do not have CHD. Dr. Stare of the Harvard School of Public Health studied the diets and heart histories of paired Irish brothers, one of whom remained in Ireland eating his high cholesterol diet while the other had emigrated to the US. The US brother ate less cholesterol but had *more* CHD.

One would think that this would cause one to lose faith in the cholesterol theory of CHD. But no, Dr. Stare saved the theory by simply assuming Ireland had less stress than the US and that this caused the unexpected results. Thus was born the Stress Theory of coronary heart disease. Though the stress theory has merit, Dr. Stare nevertheless persisted in espousing the cholesterol theory.

Another blow to the cholesterol theory was struck when it was found that serum cholesterol levels in people over age 65 had no discernible effect on one's subsequent health or risk of CHD. Hardline cholesterol proponents argue that, by age 65, the damage is done. The truth is, however, that no study has found that attempts to lower the cholesterol level after age 65 has any value whatsoever.

THE MORE LIKELY CAUSES OF CHD

1. As we have discussed earlier, proper nutrition is paramount. The great majority of our bodies' cholesterol is synthesized in the liver from sugars and refined starches, and only about 15% from dietary fat. Excess calories alone, regardless of type, will increases cholesterol synthesis. Certain fats such as cows' milk fat and "feedlot" meat fat do not fit all that well in our metabolic pathways and end up as LDL-cholesterol which is less soluble in blood and more likely to become sediment that clogs our arteries. In addition, hydrogenated fats and commercial salad oils (pressed from seeds) become altered in the process (to trans-fatty acids) and no longer fit our metabolic pathways and, thus, become atherogenic. Cutting down on sugar and refined starches will reduce cholesterol synthesis. It's that simple. Our diet should consist of fresh vegetables, legumes, whole grains, fruit, fish, shell fish, fowl, olive or flax-seed oil, and eggs are OK. We must strictly avoid homogenized milk, dairy fats, processed foods, processed oils (no matter how wholesome they were prior to processing), sweets and pastries, refined flour (pancakes, etc.), fatty meats, and excess calories in general.

2. Other nutritional factors are important, also. Hypomagnesia (low magnesium level) contributes to cardiovascular mortality. Magnesium protects against the myocardial excitability that occurs af-

ter a myocardial infarction. Intravenous magnesium, given at the time of the infarction, significantly reduces the risk of death. The cardiomyopathy of alcoholics is consistently related to hypomagnesia of myocardial cells. Our modern diet is low in magnesium and this is a factor in deaths due to heart attacks. Magnesium is plentiful in whole grains, legumes, and other vegetables. Serum magnesium level is <u>not</u> an accurate indicator of cellular magnesium: red blood cell magnesium level is a far better test.

Low serum levels of vitamins E and C and other antioxidants correlate with increased likelihood of oxidation reactions, particularly of LDL-cholesterol, the chief agent of atherogenesis. As a single factor, the taking of vitamin E supplements reduced CHD deaths by 40-60% in both men and women, according to recent studies.

Low dietary fiber correlates with higher serum cholesterol levels and increased risk of cardiac disease. (See chapter 5.)

3. Exercise is important. It uses up extra calories we eat. During our youth, exercise serves to develop larger arteries supplying the heart and other muscles. Larger arteries can tolerate a limited accumulation of atherogenic plaques without becoming clogged. Also, aerobic exercise "burns off" fats.

4. What about stress? Yes, stress is important but it is stress of a slightly different nature than you might at first think. It is the stress of loneliness and alienation. In previous ages, people enjoyed the allegiance and support of family or clan and the comfort of stable expectations. In "modern" society we have lost these health-giving support mechanisms. Our job security is fragile, our families fragmented, our cities are full of strangers, our basic values are questioned, and we feel apart, alone, and afraid. In reaction, we futilely seek material gain, join odd clubs and illusionary spiritual movements, and our young become gang members. Our sense of place in the general scheme of things has evaporated in a melange of conflicting cultures and the impermanence of our roles. That is the discontent that literally tears at one's heart and soul.

5. Hormone balance is important to vascular spasm. When vas-

cular spasm involves the arterioles (the tiny artery branches just before the blood flow enters the capillaries), it creates a resistance in the circulatory system that raises blood pressure. When it happens in coronary arteries, it can cause a heart attack. In males, most heart attacks are associated with almost complete cholesterol blockage of coronary arteries. In females, usually there is less of this cholesterol plaque in their coronary arteries. Yet, when females have a heart attack, it is more likely to be lethal. Heart attacks prior to menopause are rare. After menopause, the incidence of heart attack deaths in women rises so that the ultimate incidence approaches that of males. Because of this, it has been thought that estrogen protects against coronary spasm. However, tests by Dr. Kent Hermsmeyer & colleagues at the Oregon Regional Primate Research Center (U. of Oregon) in which artery spasm is induced in Rhesus monkeys after ovariectomy find that estrogen (Premarin) plus progesterone (in normal physiologic doses) prevents coronary artery spasm whereas estrogen plus synthetic progestins (Provera) leads to unremitting and lethal coronary spasm. In that manner, a partial artery blockage by cholesterol plaque becomes a complete blockage when the artery goes into spasm, thus causing death.

In addition, studies by Cheng and colleagues (J Clin Endo & Metab 1999; 64: 265-271) report two protective antiatherogenic effects of progesterone: (1) inhibition of cholesteryl ester synthesis; and (2) blocking of cortisol-induced cholesterol accumulation in arteries. These findings indicate that lack of progesterone or the use of synthetic progestins may be major factors in the incidence of heart disease deaths in postmenopausal women. Yet, at this date, these factors are totally ignored by cardiologists.

6. Anabolic-catabolic balance is also important. Dr. Jens Moller, of Copenhagen, spent a lifetime studying and treating vascular diseases. He found that testosterone was the most potent medicine he could give to reverse the ravages of severe vascular disease (atherogenesis, CHD), even diabetic gangrene. From this he developed the theory of balance between anabolic and catabolic metabolism. Anabolic metabolism builds and repairs tissue, and

creates energy for life's processes. Catabolic metabolism tears apart normal tissues and speeds up the aging process. He demonstrated that serum cholesterol is merely a marker for metabolic imbalance created by excessive catabolic metabolism and deficient anabolic metabolism. Attempts to lower cholesterol by diet or drugs do little to slow or reverse atherogenesis. The best treatment is to restore anabolic metabolism. In this balancing act, testosterone is the most potent anabolic hormone and cortisol is the most potent catabolic hormone. We now know that progesterone is also an anabolic hormone. Dr. Moller pointed out that stress generally leads to increased cortisol production. Therefore, while maintaining good levels of testosterone in males and/or progesterone in females, we should also strive to reduce stress.

As in the case of Dr. McCully (see #9 below), Dr. Moller garnered more criticism than plaudits despite his well-documented research. Dr. Moller was president of the European Organization for the Control of Circulatory Diseases and his book, *Cholesterol*, was published by Springer-Verlag in 1987. Though well known in Scandinavian countries, his work has been essentially ignored in the US. Dr. Shippen, in his book, *The Testosterone Syndrome*, recalls that his father, also a physician, used to tell him that "Physicians tend to be down on what they're not up on."

7. The role of alcohol is enigmatic. Too much alcohol can ruin the liver and be toxic to heart muscle cells. There is some question about whether or not the toxicity is due to alcohol alone or to alcohol in the presence of inadequate nutrition (especially magnesium and thiamine). Good epidemiologic studies, however, show that alcohol in moderation has a beneficial effect on HDL-cholesterol ratios, even a bit better than total abstinence. It appears that 2-4 oz. of hard liquor a day, or its equivalent in wine, is associated with the best cholesterol ratios. More recent studies in France where boys at age ten quit drinking milk and switch to watered red wine and, as adults, drink wine with meals, indicate that red wine may be especially protective. The fact that the annual per capita sugar consumption in France is only five lbs and in the US it is 90 lbs may also play a role here.

8. The role of cigarette smoking is not enigmatic; there is little doubt it increases CHD. Chemicals (e.g., benzo[a]pyrene) in cigarette smoke absorb into the blood stream where they are inflammatory to endothelial cells leading to cholesterol deposition and plaque formation. It should not be surprising to learn that not only coronary arteries are harmed in this manner but also carotid arteries that carry blood to the brain. Thus, early strokes are a significant cigarette smoking risk. In addition, cigarette-induced lung damage (emphysema) reduces adequate ventilation and the exchange of carbon dioxide and oxygen.

9. The role of homocysteine is also important. Homocysteine is a waste product of methionine (a sulfur-containing amino acid) metabolism. In the metabolism and urinary excretion of methionine, homocysteine is a temporary intermediary product. Over 25 years ago, Dr. Kilmer McCully, a Harvard professor of pathology, observed that children with a particular genetic defect accumulated homocysteine and developed extensive plaque formation in their arteries, leading to heart attacks and strokes. In examining adults, Dr. McCully found that people differ in their efficiency in metabolizing homocysteine to its final product prior to excretion in urine. Those with relatively high homocysteine blood or urine levels were also more at risk of developing arterial plaque and consequent heart disease and strokes. This problem afflicts approximately 15% of people. The damaging effect of high homocysteine levels is considerably more potent than that due to elevated cholesterol levels.

The enzymes that aid in the proper metabolization of homocysteine utilize vitamins B12, folic acid, and B6. Supplementation of these vitamins increases the efficiency of the enzymatic steps that reduce homocysteine levels. The Harvard Nurses Questionnaire study found that women who routinely use these vitamins, especially folic acid, as supplements were about 50% less likely to suffer heart attacks. For people found to have higher than normal homocysteine levels, treatment should include limitation of methionine-containing food (meat, for instance), and oral supplementation of B12 (1 mg), folic acid (800 mcg [8 mg]), and B6 (50 mg). It may be helpful to reflect on the fact that the same studies that showed a correlation of increased risk of CHD with meat consumption does not necessarily imply that the cause is the meat fat; it just as well can mean that the cause is a methionine metabolism defect in quite a number of people.

Dr. McCully's discovery of the homocysteine problem and the doubt he raised concerning the cholesterol theory was not only largely ignored for a quarter century and but he was demoted at Harvard. Now, however, his findings have been vindicated. Sadly, this example of blind neglect by conventional medicine and career damage to scientists going against the stream is not rare in medical history.

10. Hypertension increases the work load of the heart and, thereby, the risk of earlier CHD and stroke. Here again, stress plays an important role in the etiology of hypertension. See chapter 10 for prevention of hypertension.

11. The prostaglandin balance is important. Prostaglandin hormones modulate inflammation. One set increases inflammation and the other decreases it. The pro-inflammatory set increases vasoconstriction, platelet aggregation, cellular proliferation, and suppresses the immune system. The anti-inflammatory set causes vasodilation, inhibits platelet aggregation, controls cell proliferation, and enhances the immune system. This, in turn, is mediated by fats we eat. Omega-3 and Omega-6 fatty acids are especially important to prostaglandin balance. The reader is encouraged to read *The Anti-Aging Zone* by Barry Sears, PhD, and *Fats that Heal, Fats that Kill* by Udo Erasmus, PhD, for their well-referenced reviews of this complex subject.

Here, as elsewhere, prevention is more important than any treatment that can be given later. The earlier one learns to follow a proper diet, to exercise, and to regain a healthy 'joie de vivre', the better are the chances that CHD will be prevented. Do not wait until you find yourself in some coronary care unit before you elect to learn these lessons.

The range of nutrients that may lower CHD risk is quite extensive. For the readers' interest, see the following list. Do not fall into the trap in thinking that any specific factor is the "right" factor. They probably all contribute in varying degrees and in various ways to protection against CHD.

Vitamin C   helps lower serum cholesterol and prevent cholesterol oxidation.

Vitamin E   helps prevent cholesterol oxidation, decreases tendency of arterial wall plaque formation.

Vitamin A   also an antioxidant, strengthens cell membranes, lowers risk of myocardial infarction and stroke.

Vitamin B6   aids in the proper urinary excretion of homocysteine.

Folic Acid   also aids in the proper urinary excretion of homocysteine.

Vitamin B12   also aids in the proper metabolism of methionine and homocysteine.

Zinc   facilitates utilization of vitamin A.

Magnesium   protects against increased myocardial excitability especially in the event of a myocardial infarction.

Linoleic Acid (Omega-6) one of the essential fatty acids, poorly supplied by our processed food diet. Suppresses inflammation and contributes to cell repair. Necessary for prostaglandin hormone synthesis. Found in plant seed oils (e.g., evening primrose).

Alpha-Linolenic Acid (Omega-3) - the second essential fatty acid. It contributes to repair of endothelial

inflammation and reduces platelet aggregation. Also necessary for prostaglandin hormone synthesis. Found in certain seed oils
such as flaxseed oil.

Eicosapentanoic Acid (EPA - another Omega-3 fatty acid) –
also involved in prostaglandin hormone
processes with actions similar to above.
Found primarily in fish oils.

Docosahexanoic Acid (DHA- another Omega-3 fatty acid) -
similar to EPA above. Also found in fish oils.

Alcohol   At doses of 2-4 oz/day, significantly reduces
incidence of heart disease. Mechanism of
action still obscure.

Red Wine   Contains quinones that are antioxidants that
lower cholesterol and prevent plaque accumulation. Dose 8-16 oz/day.

Testosterone supplementation helps restore good anabolic
effect (see #4 above).

Progesterone supplementation helps restore good anabolic
effect (see #4 above).

This list above may appear daunting. It is important to note,
however, that it is better to be happy with a fairly good diet than to
be tense and obsessed seeking a perfect one. In simple terms, eat
sparingly, choose a varied diet of fresh and relatively unprocessed
vegetables, legumes, and fruit of all sorts, plus smaller amounts of
organic meat and fish, add the important antioxidants, and avoid
sugar and refined carbohydrates. There is no single diet that is perfect for all. We all differ in our metabolic needs. Moderation is a concept not to be ignored. Bon appetit!

The role of estrogen is widely touted to reduce cardiovascular
disease. This is based on circumstantial evidence. The real question
is – how much estrogen is enough? Women continue to make

estrogen after menopause in their body fat. If it is sufficient, why add more? Several good studies, including the long-running Framingham Study, find no reduction of cardiac disease in estrogen-using postmenopausal women compared to controls, nor did a 5-year double blind, placebo-controlled, randomized study comparing Premarin and Provera users with placebo controls (*JAMA*, 1998;280:605-613.)

WARNING! Cigarette smoking is toxic to endothelial cells and promotes atherosclerosis. It probably causes more heart and stroke deaths than lung cancer and emphysema deaths.

WHAT ABOUT CHOLESTEROL LOWERING DRUGS?

When confronted by patients with elevated cholesterol, contemporary physicians will often advise a "low cholesterol" diet. This diet, as recommended by the pharmaceutical industry and the American Heart Association, is likely to fail since it ignores the relevance of sugars, refined starches, and trans-fatty acids. When it fails, the physician feels obliged to prescribe one or another of the cholesterol lowering drugs. Physicians are deluged with pharmaceutical ads that claim these drugs reduce the incidence of heart deaths. Having not read the primary research himself, the physician is unaware that these drugs are uniformly correlated with higher total deaths from all causes, i.e., in randomized primary prevention trials, the patients placed on the drugs suffered a higher death rate than the control patients who were given placebo. A review of the available six studies follows:

CHOLESTEROL REDUCTION TRIALS: COMPARISON OF TOTAL MORTALITY RESULTS

Six randomized primary prevention trials of cholesterol reduction, two using diet and four using drugs, found a 7% increase in net mortality in the treated groups over controls.

Source	Study Group	# Deaths	# Subjects	Risk Ratio
Dayton et al,	Diet	117	424	1.21
1969	Control	96	422	
Franz et al,	Diet	208	4541	1.07
1989	Control	194	4516	
WHO Cooperative	Clofibrate	239	5331	1.33
Trial, 1980	Control	179	5296	
Dorr et al,	Colestipol	18	1149	1.04
1978	Control	17	1129	
Lipid Research	Cholestyramine	38	1906	1.15
Program, 1984	Control	33	1900	
Frick et al,	Gemfibrozil	43	2051	1.58
1990	Control	27	2030	

In all trials, despite a modest decrease in cardiac deaths, total mortality was higher in the treated groups than in the controls. (source: *JAMA*, 1 Jan 1992;627:100)

These drugs lower cholesterol (1) by binding to fats such that their absorption in the gut is prevented or (2) by increasing biliary excretion of cholesterol and fats, both of which result in a greater amount of fat entering the colon where bacteria await to make them rancid. This, as one might imagine, leads to symptoms of indigestion, gas, and the metabolic results of the rancid fats. Side effects are numerous and undesirable. The higher death rates are due, in part, to an increase in accident fatalities, manslaughter and suicide, and, possibly colon cancer in the future. In addition, the drugs are expensive.

Not surprisingly, most physicians have now abandoned these particular cholesterol-lowering drugs and opted for newer entrants in the field, (e.g., lovastatin [trade name Mevacor]), which work in a different manner: they interrupt the synthesis of cholesterol at an early step in the process. The fate of products accumulating as a result of this interruption is presently unknown. Also unknown are the long term effects. These drugs have become the #1 cholesterol-lowering drug class, and pharmaceutical companies are bringing out similar products with which to compete for the market. It does appear to lower CHD deaths more effectively than earlier drugs. Interestingly, however, its benefits seem to be unrelated to initial cholesterol levels. Thus, some scientists suspect that its cardio-protective effects stem from a different mechanism of action, still unknown.

A BETTER WAY

How much better it would be if doctors could teach their patients the right diet, create hormone balance, and reduce stress. If one were cynical, one might suspect that the futile "low cholesterol" diet as proposed by the pharmaceutical companies (and even by the Heart Association) is nothing more than a clever stratagem to induce physicians to prescribe these drugs when the diet fails.

Nutritional defenses are important. If you are young and found to have an elevated cholesterol level with an undesirably low HDL-cholesterol and your doctor does not recommend the nutritional defenses as outlined in the pages above, it might be wise to find a doctor who will. At the present time, there exists no valid reason to accept the known increased risks of death offered by drugs.

A case in point is Dr. Dean Ornish, of the University of California, San Francisco, School of Medicine, who has shown that diet and stress reduction not only lowers cholesterol but *reverses atherosclerosis within the coronary arteries*. CHD is not due to Mevacor deficiency; it is a metabolic disease associated with an inappropriate diet, hormone imbalance, and excess stress. Does it not seem obvious that correction of these problems is the direction one should take to pursue one's goal of optimal health?

In July 1993, the nation's largest health insurer, Mutual of Omaha, recognized Dr. Ornish's atherosclerosis treatment program as reimbursable. His program of nutrition, exercise, and stress reduction instruction is just as effective but is only one-tenth the cost of conventional medical care. The contemporary interventionist techniques such as coronary bypass surgery - our nation's No. 1 medical expense - provides a stopgap amelioration of the coronary problem but does nothing to prevent its recurrence.

An interesting question that should be asked is - which is more "radical"?

a) Cutting open a patient's chest and implanting a leg vein to replace a coronary artery or,

b) Putting the patient on a good diet, get his/her hormone balance in order, teach stress reduction techniques, encourage moderate exercise and enroll in a support group to keep him/her on track with a new life style.

Most, one would hope, would opt for the latter. This is the type of preventive medicine that our doctors should learn if they are to properly serve their patients. Think of the savings in terms of health and health costs when prevention becomes the norm.

SUMMARY GUIDELINE FOR PREVENTION OF ATHEROSCLEROSIS

- Have the right grandparents.

- Do a lot of running and other good exercise while young.

- Remain slim.

- Never smoke cigarettes.

- Avoid sugars, pastries, refined starches of any kind. Whole grains are OK.

- Avoid dairy fats (after puberty), and "feed lot fats."

- Eat lots of fresh vegetables; make them 75-80% of your diet.

- Do not be afraid of fish, shellfish, olive oil, or eggs.

- Avoid commercial pressed oils from nuts and seeds; avoid margarine.

- A little butter with vegetables is OK.

- Continue exercise throughout life.

- Take "breaks" from stress, develop a sense of humor, and smell the roses.

- Correct hormone balance with testosterone (in males) or progesterone (in females).

- A modest intake of alcohol is OK as far as your arteries are concerned.

- In supermarkets, stick to the walls; avoid all center aisles.

SELF QUIZ

1. Coronary atherosclerosis, the leading cause of death in the US, has been common since 1850. True or False?

2. The cause of this disease, i.e., cholesterol accumulation in the coronary arteries, is due to dietary cholesterol. True or False?

3. Serum cholesterol can be divided into two parts: high density lipoprotein (HDL) and low density lipoprotein (LDL). Which one is protective?

4. Diet has little or no effect on our blood cholesterol. True or False?

5. Give two examples of foods that are likely to raise one's cholesterol. _____ and _____.

6. Eggs contain approximately 200 mg of cholesterol in their yolks. Yet, eating six eggs a week is perfectly all right. True or False?

7. French males quit drinking milk at age 8-10 years and switch to watered red wine. They have a low incidence of heart disease. Do you think this is due to (a) quitting milk, (b) drinking red wine, (c) both, or (4) neither?

8. According to the WHO, per capita sugar consumption in the US is 90 lb per year and in France it is 5 lbs per year. True or False?

9. When tested, margarine is found safer to eat than butter. True or False?

10. Certain medications are prescribed for lowering cholesterol. When these are tested by controlled studies, they actually *increase* subsequent mortality rates, compared to control patients. True or False?

Answers can be found on page 194.

CHAPTER TEN
ARTERIOSCLEROSIS
AND HYPERTENSION

Arteriosclerosis and hypertension are often interrelated. Arteriosclerosis (literally: hardening of the arteries) refers to a thickening and hardening of the artery walls. It is thought to occur, in most instances, due to (1) chronic wear and tear of the arteries in response to the pounding pressure of the blood being pushed through them by the heart and to (2) deterioration in the elasticity of arterial wall connective tissue, a defect probably related to lack of antioxidants vitamins C and E and other dietary or environmental factors.

With each heartbeat, a surge of blood is pushed out into the arteries by contraction of the left cardiac ventricle (systole). The arteries receiving this surge of blood expand from the pressure of the surge and then, when the heart is briefly resting (during diastole) to receive blood being brought to it by the veins, contract again to their normal caliber. Thus, the pressure within the arteries does not fall to zero in the interval between beats. If the arteries were like water pipes and did not have this elastic quality, the peak blood pressure with each heartbeat would be very high indeed. For many years, this marvelous elasticity of the arteries preserves a relatively smooth blood flow throughout the vascular system. In time, however, a certain thickening and stiffness of artery walls does occur and thus we see that, with age, a person's "blood pressure" tends to appear to rise. Older doctors commonly say that the systolic blood pressure can be considered normal if it does not exceed 100 + age of the patient and the diastolic pressure does not exceed 94 mm Hg.

Other factors can cause thickening and hardening of one's arteries. This happens more often to cigarette smokers, probably due to toxic ingredients in cigarette smoke taken up by the arteries through the lungs and mucosa of the mouth and throat. Rarely, there also is a genetic factor, which predisposes one to serious arterial wall thickening (Buerger's disease). There also are important dietary factors, which will be discussed below.

By experience it is evident that chronic stress can cause hypertension. This effect involves two related mechanisms: (1) more forceful heart contractions under stress and (2) stress-related contraction of arterioles (the very tiny artery branches that immediately precede the capillary beds) increasing the resistance to the flow of blood. It can be shown that certain kinds of stress induced in test animals do lead to hypertension. In humans, it is quite easy to demonstrate stress-induced hypertension, at least initially. But often this is found to be transient as humans have the ability to adapt to conditions that are initially stressful. Life, however, is complex and may bring chronic recurring episodes of stress that will, in susceptible persons, lead to increased wear and tear on the arteries which causes arteriosclerosis and creates a vicious cycle in which arterial hardening causes increased hypertension and the hypertension causes more arterial damage. To prevent fixed hypertension (and the consequent arteriosclerosis), it is important to find the hypertension and treat it properly before more damage is done.

Epidemiologic studies clearly demonstrate that hypertension is common in some populations and almost non-existent in others, and that the difference is due to diet. This dietary difference concerns the relative intake of sodium and potassium. As we discussed earlier, sodium is the predominant electrolyte of extracellular fluid while potassium and magnesium are the predominant electrolytes of fluid within our cells. This separation is maintained by sodium and potassium biochemical "pumps" within the cell membrane; one "pump" system keeping sodium out and another one keeping potassium in. Intracellular potassium concentration is approximately 18 times that of the blood serum.

Cell membrane "pumps" evolved throughout millions of years in an environment in which the ratio of dietary sodium and potassium was one part sodium for every 20-200 parts potassium, which is the usual ratio of these two minerals in all natural foods. This type of diet is typical of "undeveloped" countries where hypertension is rare. In industrialized societies, the diet consists largely of processed foods in which raw foods are cooked and then canned for longer shelf life and distribution through our super markets. Both these minerals are water-soluble and are lost when the cooking water is discarded prior to canning. With the minerals gone, the taste is flat. Food processors, therefore, customarily add sodium chloride (i.e., "salt") to restore a "zesty" taste. The ratio of sodium: potassium is thus changed from 1:100 to 100:1. This reversal of the normal "salt" ratio is the main cause of what doctors call "essential hypertension." The excess sodium places a great burden on the body in trying to get rid of it and the deficiency of potassium weakens all cells, especially their membrane "pumps."

In this regard, the usual blood tests will not reveal this imbalance as our homeostatic mechanisms will maintain the usual serum levels at the expense of the potassium usually present within the cells. Large epidemiologic studies find this dietary sodium: potassium reversal is correlated not only with hypertension but also with higher incidence of cancer, hemorrhoids, weakness, headaches, aging, heart disease, and earlier death. Yet this important relationship is largely unrecognized in our society. We seem inextricably bound to a reliance on processed foods.

The chart below indicates the relative content of sodium and potassium in natural foods.

Relative content of sodium and potassium in natural foods:		
Food type	Sodium/Potassium ratio	Average
Vegetables	range: 1/10 to 1/200	1/30
Fruit	range: 1/50 to 1/250	1/100
Nuts	range: 1/50 to 1/400	1/200
Grains/cereals	range: 1/100 to 1/200	1/150
Meats	range: 1/3 to 1/6	1/5
Fish	range: 1/4 to 1/8	1/5

Processing of food changes drastically the content of sodium and potassium. The following chart of some typical examples illustrates the great change in the ratio of sodium to potassium when food is cooked and salt is added.

Content of Sodium (Na) and Potassium (K) in raw and processed (canned) foods:				
Food type	Raw food Na & K		Processed food Na & K	
Beans, green - 1/2 cup	7 mg	243 mg	270 mg	104 mg
Peas - 1/2 cup	1 mg	211 mg	117 mg	72 mg
Tomatoes, raw	3 mg	244 mg	130 mg	217 mg
Vegetable beef soup	30 mg	300 mg	1230 mg	100 mg
Blueberry muffin			253 mg	48 mg
Average "TV" dinner			1200 mg	NR

Our sodium intake is, for the most part, hidden from our awareness. Most people do not realize that our diet often provides 8-10,000 mg of sodium per day, whereas our bodies only need about 1500 mg per day. We have no warning lights on our dashboards to tell us that we are overdosed with sodium and very deficient in potassium. (Hypertension causes no symptoms until the problem is advanced and some catastrophe such as a stroke occurs. In the US, 30% of adults are found to be hypertensive and over 70% of us will eventually have hypertension.) The average person is unaware that foods with excess sodium and deficient potassium include bread, cereals, and canned vegetables, especially the canned soups. (Buying "low sodium" soup is a waste of time because it still lacks potassium, and has little or no taste.) Salami, bologna, and most sausages are heavily salted as a means of preserving them, a practice of necessity before the days of refrigeration. Our breads and breakfast rolls are made with baking powder and, often, baking soda, both of which contain sodium bicarbonate. Green vegetables sold as frozen are laced with sodium benzoate to enhance the green color. The addition of the sodium from the salt shaker is, in fact, only a minor factor. If a person eats only fresh foods, he/she can use the salt shaker in moderation without fear.

Further, it is well established that women given hormonal therapy (contraceptive pills and postmenopausal hormone replacement) using synthetic hormone substitutes for estrogen and progesterone may develop hypertension. This is due to a side effect of these synthetic analogues of the natural hormones in which renin substrate and aldosterone excretion rate are abnormally elevated thus leading to hypertension. Fortunately, this side-effect will subside in 1-7 months after discontinuing the synthetic hormones.

TREATMENT OF HYPERTENSION

Many medications exist for treating hypertension. None should be used until proper dietary changes have been made. When the role of sodium and potassium is understood in relation to the foods we eat and appropriate changes made, hypertension, if caught early, usually clears. Obesity, per se, does not cause hypertension or arteriosclerosis. The proper dietary change should focus on reducing sodium and restoring the proper intake of potassium. Only if that fails should one turn to medications for treating hypertension.

These drugs work in one of several ways. Some (e.g., propranolol and other beta blockers) will partially weaken the force of the heart beat to reduce the surge of blood with each beat. Others (e.g., hydralazine) partially paralyze the muscles at various sites within the arterial system so that our arteries become more dilated and allow a larger vascular bed for the push of the blood but can cause *orthostatic hypotension*, i.e., fainting when getting up from a prone or sitting position. Diuretics (e.g., furosemide or hydro-chlorthiazide) trick the kidneys into making more urine than usual, thus reducing the watery component of our blood volume. Calcium channel blockers prevent rapid smooth muscle contraction. Others (e.g., captopril) inhibit angiotensin converting enzyme; and still others (methyldopa or clonidine) block stress centers in the brain or impair the nerves that carry stress messages to arteries. All of these drugs have potentially dangerous side effects. The advantage of using the dietary approach should be obvious.

Advice to patients of physicians: Do not rely on blood pressure measurements taken in the doctor's office; they are often higher than when you are at home. Whatever drug is prescribed, the dosage may be higher than needed and you will experience hypotension (low blood pressure) when at home. Obtain a blood pressure meter for home use and learn how to use it. Keep a record and show your doctor when you see him/her. It might help prevent overdosing.

Advice to elderly patients: Antihypertensive drugs have side effects that are especially dangerous for frail patients. The risk of dangerous drug side effects may be greater than the potential benefit of the drug. Also, the effective dose may be less in an elderly person than in a young person. It is important to prevent unnecessary and/or excessive doses.

Hypertension vignette:

When I was teaching Optimal Health at the College of Marin, various members of the college teaching staff often audited my class. On one occasion, Mrs. V, an older woman who taught a class on coping with aging, happened to drop in when the topic was hypertension. This as it turned out was particularly important to her since she was being treated for hypertension and osteoporosis. Her doctor had prescribed estrogen for her. The estrogen caused ankle edema for which he had then prescribed Lasix, a calcium-losing diuretic. This accelerated her osteoporosis, leading to a higher dose of estrogen that, again, caused edema, and her Lasix dose was increased. On hearing of the sodium/potassium balance problem and the importance of avoiding canned food, she went home and threw out all her canned food. Within two weeks both her edema and hypertension were gone. She sent me a nice note to read to the class, reporting that she lost 12 lbs of water on a diet of fresh, unprocessed vegetables, used low-dose estrogen and no diuretics, and was feeling fine.

The concept is simple, its application is easy, and vindication is sweet.

SELF QUIZ

1. In America, 30% of adults are hypertensive and 70% of us will eventually be treated for hypertension; yet, in other cultures, hypertension is rare. The difference is due to (a) genetics, (b) diet, or (c) stress. Pick one

2. In treating hypertension, the most important thing is to find the best drug to get the blood pressure back to normal. True or False?

3. Sodium and potassium are two essential minerals. In unprocessed foods, _____ is much more abundant than _____, whereas in processed foods, the ratio is frequently reversed.

4. When grocery shopping, choose those foods labeled "low sodium." True or False?

5. Hardening of the arteries causes hypertension. True or False?

6. Hypertension causes hardening of the arteries. True or False?

7. In the US, daily dietary sodium often ranges from 8000-10,000 mg/day. True or False?

8. Typical daily sodium requirement is 1500 mg/day. True or False?

9. A person can tell by how he feels if he has hypertension. True or False?

10. Development of hypertension has little to do with vitamin C or vitamin E. True or False?

Answers can be found on page 194.

CHAPTER ELEVEN
CANCER

Cancer refers to the abnormal growth of cells in our bodies suffi-cient to kill us if left untreated. All cancer originates as a change of a normal cell. Three characteristics distinguish cancer cells from nor-mal cells. They are (1) an <u>increased</u> rate of multiplication, (2) a <u>loss</u> of differentiation, and (3) slowing of apoptosis (normal cell death). As we have previously stated, most body cells replicate themselves continually at a rate that is synchronous with normal growth and repair. Each cell contains a full complement (with the exception of ova and sperm) of chromosomes; yet each develops in a manner specific for its purpose in the body. When it becomes a cancer cell it multiplies faster than it should and loses its normal differentiation. Compared to normal cells, a cancer is a more primitive cell, growing in a manner more avaricious than the normal cell from whence it came.

Apoptosis (literally a "falling away") has emerged as a major fac-tor in understanding and possibly preventing cancer. Normal cells all (except brain and muscle cells) have an inherent life span; they are internally programmed to die at a given time, to be replaced by new healthier cells constantly being made. It is the normal process of renewing health and the body. A slowing of apoptosis in a given cell is the hallmark of a cancer cell. Apoptosis is controlled by spe-cific genes. Any gene mutation that causes a delay of normal apoptosis leads eventually to cancer. Prevention of altered apoptosis is now the leading candidate for cancer prevention. A more com-plete explanation of apoptosis follows below.

At present, annual cancer mortality in the US is approximately 500,000, second only to heart disease (734,000), and accounts for 23% of total deaths. Now, in 1999, the incidence of cancer deaths has risen so that one out of three of us will die of cancer. Among men, the top three cancer types causing death are lung, prostate, and colon/rectum, accounting for 57% of all male cancer deaths. Among women, the top three are lung, breast, and colon/rectum, accounting for 51% of all female cancer deaths.

It is interesting to note that only recently has the US cancer establishment recognized the importance of diet in relation to cancer. It is now generally admitted that at least 35% of our cancer results from improper diet. Chances are the correlation is considerably higher than that. Yet, in 1993, for example, the proportion of US cancer research funding budgeted for nutritional research was only 5%.

CAUSES OF CANCER

Cell growth and replication are determined by DNA (i.e., chromosomal) messages. The *genetic* theory proposes that the cancer cell is a product of DNA damage induced by radiation, viruses, or toxins. As one progresses through life, the accumulated bits of damage that occur to a cell's chromosomes gradually increase over time. Thus, the incidence of cancer increases with age. It is generally thought that, for a cell to become cancerous, five or more gene sites must be damaged. Healthy chromosomes are endowed with gene repair mechanisms, the loss of which will predispose one to cancer risk.

A more recent theory holds that certain toxic environments within the cell can stimulate a latent ability of otherwise undamaged chromosomes to switch to this more primitive mode in response to the *epigenetic* threat. This latter theory suggests that correction of the cellular environment may lead to successful non-toxic treatment (or prevention, at least) of cancer.

Evidence against the genetic theory and/or in favor of the epigenetic theory:

A. Under the same risk exposure, only some people develop cancer.

B. Under similar exposure to known carcinogens, different individuals develop cancer at different tissue sites.

C. In animals (e.g., hamsters) exposed to known carcinogens, cancer can be prevented by agents such as carotenes , vitamin A, or vitamin C, etc.

D. In cell culture tests, cancers induced by known carcinogens can be reversed and eliminated by improving the nutrient quality of the cell culture.

E. In humans with advanced cancer, survival time is often increased by adequate vitamin C.

F. Similarly, changes in patient attitude may extend survival time.

G. In humans, "spontaneous" remissions and apparent cures may result simply from dietary changes.

Cancer cells are quite difficult to kill, compared to normal cells. Our immune system, which is so effective against foreign invaders, does not recognize cancer cells as targets for attack because their cell membranes remain quite normal. Our usual treatments are surgery, radiation, or toxic chemicals and are really not very effective. If the cancer cell mass is confined, surgery can remove it or radiation can kill it but both often carry quite serious potential destructive consequences. Chemotherapy refers to the use of drugs which mimic (but not well enough to suffice for) the molecules from which multiplying cells construct their new DNA. Since the cancer cells multiply faster than normal cells, they utilize more of these abnormal molecules and thus lose their ability to multiply. The trick is to give enough to kill off a large number of cancer cells without killing too many normal cells or killing the patient. Certain cancers such as childhood leukemia or Hodgkin's lymphoma are quite amenable to therapy, possibly because their cause is more likely to be viral and/or because adequate DNA repair mechanisms are still intact. Our past attempts to kill cancer cells by surgery, chemotherapy, and/or radiation have not succeeded in lowering cancer mortality in the majority of cancers, however. Modulation of apoptosis appears to be more promising.

THE APOPTOSIS PARADIGM

Apoptosis refers to the rate at which cells die naturally. Some refer to apoptosis as programmed cell suicide. New cells are constantly replacing all the cells of the body, except brain and muscle cells. Red blood cells, for instance, live only about 120 days, white blood cells may live only 2-3 days, and new skin cells are constantly emerging while old, dead skin cells slough off. The same is true of endocrine cells and cells lining the respiratory system and gastrointestinal system. New creation of cells means that the older cells die off. This is a natural process and essential for continued good health.

Cancer cells develop from normal cells when apoptosis is delayed for whatever reason. Normal death of cells (apoptosis) is designed into the genetic controls of the cells. Some genes, called oncogenes, slow the rate of apoptosis and, when this gene is activated in a given cell, that cell is more likely to multiply more rapidly and not die on time, and becomes a cancer cell. There are other genes that oppose oncogenes and act to prevent the conversion of a normal cell into a cancer cell. The actions of these sets of genes are modulated by a number of different factors including hormones, prostaglandins, cytokines, nutrients, and even by chemical or electromagnetic influence of neighboring cells.

The example of genes Bcl-2 and p53 illustrate this process. Gene Bcl-2 is a known oncogene, i.e., its product can cause a normal cell to become a cancer cell. Gene p53, on the other hand, opposes Bcl-2 and thereby prevents a normal cell from becoming a cancer cell. In an exquisite study at UC/Santa Barbara, Professor Bent Formby and T. S. Wiley, using breast cancer cell culture, found that estradiol activated Bcl-2, causing rapid growth of cancer cells. When progesterone was added to the cancer cell culture, gene p53 product increased, causing a slowing of cell proliferation and a return of normal apoptosis. This landmark study demonstrated several very important findings: (1) genes are modulated by hormones, (2) Bcl-2 is activated by estradiol; (3) p53 is activated by progesterone; (4) estradiol, therefore, can both initiate and promote breast cancer; (5) progesterone protects against breast cancer; and (6) that the genetic and epigenetic theories are not mutually exclusive.

The example of hormone effect on breast cancer risk is not unique. The only known cause of endometrial (uterine) cancer, for example, is estrogen unopposed by progesterone. The same is probably true of prostate cancer, also. The prostate gland is the male equivalent of the female uterus. Both developed from the same embryonic cells. Therefore, it is likely that they both respond in similar fashion to the same hormone imbalance.

In a similar vein, it is now confirmed that natural vitamin E protects against breast cancer. This means that specific nutrients are also important in preventing and treating cancer. Success in preventing and treating cancer will not come from pharmaceutical drugs, it will come from understanding the many natural factors that modulate healthy cell responses and avoiding factors that predispose normal cells to become cancer cells.

It is clear that prevention is far better than treatment. US cancer incidence is quite different from that of undeveloped cultures and the difference is in environmental causes. Undeveloped areas carry the risk of aflatoxin, for instance, a soil mold contamination that leads to liver cancer. Lung cancer is clearly related to cigarette smoking. Yet, its incidence can be reduced if one has sufficient vitamin A. Colon cancer, second only to lung cancer in men and breast cancer in women, appears to be correlated with diets high in meat and low in vitamin C and fiber. Some, but not all research suggests the correlation of breast cancer with US dietary fats and/or the xenohormones (petrochemical pesticides) they might contain. As we've seen before, life choices alter the balance between defense and risk. Seeking better treatments will not relieve the scourge of cancer; the solution is prevention.

Environmental pollution is a major cancer risk. Our personal health is intimately tied to the health of the environment. It is a serious mistake to believe that humans are separate or immune to environmental factors. Among the many good books on this subject, I recommend reading the book, *Living Downstream,* by Sandra Steingraber published in 1998 by Vintage Books.

BREAST CANCER

Cancer therapists have long claimed that earlier detection will lead to more successful therapy. This, however, depends on the cancer. It is not true of lung cancer, for instance, or cancer of the liver or pancreas. Nor, unfortunately, is it true of the time advantage gained by mammograms for detecting breast cancer. Despite the wide advertisement and use of mammograms, the death rate of breast cancer over the past 2-3 decades is essentially unchanged. While it is true that mammograms may discover breast cancer at an earlier stage than simple palpation, that time difference turns out to be of no significance in outcome. Many claim that the 5-year survival after diagnosis of breast cancer is better after mammography than after palpation diagnosis but these claims are guilty of ignoring lead-time bias. If it is true that mammography can diagnose breast cancer two years before it is found by palpation, then two years should be added to the time of survival for the patient whose breast cancer is found by palpation. The patient has, after all, enjoyed two years of life before a diagnosis that would otherwise have been made two years earlier with mammograms. When this is factored in, the survival times of breast cancer is unaffected by mammogram. Thus, it can be concluded that the 2-year advantage of mammograms is, for breast cancer, of no significance.

If a breast lump is found by palpation, it is wise to use mammography to check the other breast as breast cancer is often found in both breasts. Since cancer is due to some underlying metabolic imbalance favoring cancerous changes, it is likely that both breasts are under similar risk. Therefore, it is likely that if cancer is found in one breast, it will sooner or later show up in the other breast. Breast cancer, in some studies, is strongly correlated with a high fat diet. The standard American diet derives over 40% of its calories from fat which include not only the undesirable 'trans' forms but also is heavily contaminated with fat-soluble toxic pesticides, both of which probably contribute to the cancer risk.

The role of xenohormones (petrochemical pesticides, etc.) in breast cancer is not well understood by many. In various wildlife studies, exposure to xenohormones increases the incidence of hormone dependent cancers. (See the book, *Our Stolen Future*, by Theo Colborn.) While our exposure to these toxins is low by most standards, the fact is that xenohormone *sensitivity* is vastly greater during one's embryo stage of life when tissue differentiation is taking place. In the wildlife studies, the incidence of hormone dependent cancers is greatly increased in the offspring when exposure to xenohormones occurred during the mother's pregnancy. There is no reason to believe that the same thing doesn't happen in humans. The example of DES (diethylstilbestrol) is a case in point. When used during pregnancy, the female child is much more likely to develop vaginal or urogenital cancer later in life, just as the male child is more likely to develop prostate cancer later in life. DES and similar synthetic estrogens are commonly used as "growth factors" in animals destined for meat production. These petrochemical estrogens are fat soluble and non-biodegradable and not easily avoided.

The role of hormone balancing is crucial in breast and prostate cancer. At a symposium sponsored by the National Cancer Institute (NCI) in March 1998, speakers from prestigious cancer research centers around the world presented studies showing that estradiol and estrone can follow metabolic pathways leading to gene mutations and cancer of both breast and prostate. As described above, Formby and Wiley showed that apoptosis is modulated by estradiol and progesterone balance. When estradiol is dominant, apoptosis slows and normal cells become cancer cells. When appropriate progesterone is present, apoptosis rates return to normal and the cancer risk is decreased.

In this regard, it is important to know that, among women in the industrialized world, progesterone production declines 15 or more years before menopause, a condition that creates estrogen dominance. Since it takes 8-10 years for a developing breast cancer to become clinically evident, it is not surprising that breast cancer appears so often in women in their 30s and 40s.

As with most cancers, the clues to proper treatment will be found in the etiology or causal factors of the cancer. In addition to dietary fat and its load of toxic undesirable contaminants, physicians still rarely consider the question of female hormones. Meta-analysis of earlier studies supported (but did not prove) the theory that estrogen may be a factor in causing breast cancer. A listing of some of the clues follows:

1. Pregnancy occurring before age 25-30 has a protective effect.

2. Only the first, full-term, early pregnancy conveys protection. Women having their first pregnancies before age 18 have approximately 1/3 the risk of women bearing their first child after age 35. Interrupted pregnancies (spontaneous or induced abortions) do not afford protection and may, in fact, increase the risk.

3. Women without children are at a higher risk than are women with one or more children.

4. In women subjected to oophorectomy (removal of both ovaries) prior to age 40, their risk of breast cancer is significantly reduced.

5. Protective effects of early oophorectomy are negated by administration of estrogen.

6. Treatment of males with estrogen (for prostate cancer or after trans-sexual surgery) is associated with an increased risk of breast cancer.

7. Recently, industrial pollutants having estrogenic effects ("xenoestrogens") are being recognized as a pervasive environmental threat. Such agents as are found in pesticides and plastics are, at nanogram amounts, extremely potent in their ability to mimic estrogen in their effects on the body. Research strongly suggests that increased

exposure to estrogenic substances is the cause of our high incidence of breast cancer (and the cause of the falling sperm count in men).

Hormone balance is the key. Human estrogens (estradiol and estrone), when unopposed by progesterone, are fully capable of causing and promoting breast cancer. Estriol, the dominant estrogen during pregnancy, carries no risk of breast cancer. In non-pregnant women, estriol is much less stimulating to the breast than are estrone or estradiol, the estrogens that dominate during the first two weeks of regular menstrual cycles.

The protective effect of natural progesterone is suggested by the following:

1. In premenopausal women with breast cancer treated by mastectomy, those that underwent mastectomy during the latter two weeks of their menstrual cycle (when progesterone is the dominant gonadal hormone) developed significantly *fewer* late recurrences or metastases than those women whose surgery occurred during the first two weeks of their menstrual cycle (when progesterone is absent and only estrogen is being produced by the ovaries).

2. When measured prospectively, women with progesterone deficiency were found to have 5.4 times the risk of developing premenopausal breast cancer and a 10-fold increase in deaths from all malignant neoplasms compared to the women with normal progesterone levels.

3. Breast cancer cell culture studies have now shown that estrogen activates the oncogene, Bcl-2, whereas progesterone activates the cancer-protective gene, p53.

Thus, fairly substantial evidence exists to say that unopposed estrogen (i.e., the lack of progesterone) is a risk of developing breast cancer and likewise decreases survival time after treatment. This evidence suggests that, in addition to the usual nutritional defenses, progesterone's cancer-protective effects should be used in the prevention and/or treatment of such cases.

PROSTATE CANCER

Prostate cancer may be the most common cancer in males. Previously, diagnosis depended on symptoms of urinary obstruction (more often due to benign prostatic hyperplasia) and palpation (by rectal exam) of a hard prostate lump, later confirmed by biopsy. Palpation of the prostate is a relatively crude diagnostic technique and will detect only those cancers that are located in the posterior aspect of the gland. It is likely that many small or more centrally located tumors are never discovered. Recently, however, the playing field has shifted. Transrectal ultrasound images now display the entire gland and are sufficiently sensitive to detect small islets of nonspecific irregular cellular clumps deep within the prostate tissue. In conjunction with the transrectal probe, multiple needle biopsies can be obtained of the suspicious areas. In this manner, small islets of prostate cancer cells that never before could have been found are now being detected.

In addition, a new screening test for prostate cancer, called the Prostate Specific Antigen (PSA) test, has been developed. This test measures, in nanograms per milliliter, the blood level of this antigen, a glycoprotein secreted by the normal prostate gland. Blood levels of PSA generally rise as men get older and after massage or manipulation of the prostate. With prostate cancer, PSA levels also usually rise. When used for detecting prostate cancer, the PSA test gives incorrect results at least 20% to 35% of the time. The test may miss detecting some prostate cancers or, if elevated, may imply cancer where none exists. Present medical technique uses the PSA test to select patients on whom to employ the transrectal ultrasound and needle biopsy tests. When used in this fashion, so-called precancerous prostate islets are found in 22% of men between the ages of 30 and 39, and cancer is detected in 41% of men between the ages of 40 and 49. The percentage of men with microscopic prostate cancer found in this manner rises with age, reaching an incidence of probably over 75-80% of men older than 75. The market for prostate cancer therapy has now increased dramatically.

The problem is that, since these microscopic cancer islets were never previously diagnosed, their natural course is unknown. It is not known, for instance, whether they will progress or remain microscopic and insignificant. Should they be treated by surgical or chemical castration, prostatectomy surgery, or radiation, or should they merely be monitored over time using the PSA test and transrectal ultrasound? In Europe, where such patients over age 70 were divided into two groups, one receiving therapy and the other merely monitored, the subsequent mortality rates were the same for the two groups; and mortality due to prostate cancer was equally low in both groups.

Ever since Dr. Charles Huggins advocated surgical castration for prostate cancer, over 50 years ago, contemporary medicine assumed that the etiology of prostate cancer was related to the male hormone, testosterone. This conclusion is now being re-evaluated. Some have suggested that the putative benefit of castration reported by Dr. Huggins may have been merely a statistical illusion created by an unrecognized mismatch of the staging of the prostate cancers being treated. Even more likely is the fact that the role of estrogen production by the testes was ignored. I suspect that low testosterone and the emergence of estrogen dominance is the true cause of prostate cancer.

Do you not find it curious that prostate cancer is unheard of during early adult life when testosterone levels are highest? Castration is not benign: since testosterone (like progesterone) activates new bone formation, its removal routinely results in osteoporosis. We should not forget that the prostate is the male equivalent of the female uterus. The only known cause of uterine cancer is unopposed estrogen. It has been a mistake, in my opinion, that progesterone has been ignored in prostate cancer research.

Prostate cancer, like many cancers, very likely develops in tissue that is deprived of essential nutrients. In this case, essential fatty acids appear to be especially important. I know of patients with biopsy-proved islets of prostate cancer who have opted for nutritional treatment using flaxseed oil (rich in essential fatty acids), zinc, vitamins C, A, and E, and selenium, and a good diet have been rewarded by a return of low PSA readings and the diminution or disappearance of their lesions on ultra-sound testing, all without losing their testosterone. Such results cause much consternation among the urologists who had predicted an early death unless treated with castration, prostate resection, chemotherapy, or radiation. The financial gain to the patients is not inconsiderable, also.

COLON/RECTAL CANCER

Colon/rectal cancer, the number two cancer in the US, is especially preventable and treatable. It is extremely rare in cultures with a high fiber/low meat diet. In addition to low fiber and high meat diet factors, colon cancer is correlated with a number of other, possibly related factors. A listing would include the following:

1. Low fiber diet, e.g., < 25-30 grams a day

2. High red meat diet

3. Prolonged G-I transit time, e.g., over 30 hours

4. Chronic over-eating resulting in a chronically food-filled colon

5. High protein diet, i.e., > 5-6 ounces a day

6. Low vitamin C (vitamin C blocks bacterial fermentation that otherwise converts excess proteins into nitrosamine, a colon cancer precursor.)

7. Elevated iron load, e.g., hemochromatosis patients

8. Trans-fatty acids

All of these potential etiologic factors could be eliminated by modest dietary changes such as choosing a diet high in fresh, unprocessed vegetables, legumes, grains, and fruit, with modest amounts of seafood and fowl, and strictly limiting red meat and deep fat frying and other sources of trans-fatty acids. It should be obvious by now to the reader that, no matter what illness is being studied, the most effective dietary advice returns to the same basic diet.

LUNG CANCER

This cancer, the nation's leader among causes of cancer deaths, occurs almost exclusively in cigarette smokers. It does little good to attempt to dissect out just what factor in cigarettes is the true cause. The best protection is to not smoke cigarettes. Undoubtedly, other factors may emerge; e.g., particulate matter from air-borne industrial waste. One particularly vicious form of lung cancer, mesothelioma, is due to microscopic asbestos fibers and, in this case, it matters very little whether the fibers were inhaled or ingested.

In addition to the avoidance of cigarette smoking, certain nutritional factors (e.g., vitamin E) are modestly protective against the development of lung cancer. This should not be construed to mean that smoking is safe if these factors are present.

Little more can be said about lung cancer. Contemporary treatments are relatively ineffective; some may induce a reduction in tumor size but cure can not be realistically anticipated.

BONE CANCER (OSTEOSARCOMA)

Despite the fact that osteosarcoma is rare (2.9 cases per million people), it is one of the principal cancers of young people. There is, moreover, an interesting lesson to learn from a look at this problem. In 1990, the results of a National Toxicology Program (NTP) fluoride/ cancer study using rats and mice showed an unexpected but statistically significant dose-related incidence of osteosarcoma in male rats. In 1991, the US Public Health Service reviewed the National Cancer Institute's epidemiology files concerning osteosarcoma in the US and found higher incidences of osteosarcoma in young males living in fluoridated communities. In 1992, the New Jersey Department of Health studied the incidence of osteosarcoma in young males living in fluoridated and unfluoridated communities in New Jersey. The study's author, Dr. P.D. Cohn, reported that the incidence of osteosarcoma in New Jersey is 6.9 times greater in fluoridated communities, compared to unfluoridated communities. Despite these findings, the US Public Health Service continues to advocate fluoridation and instead is calling for more funding to investigate the problem further.

Fluoride, it should be recalled, has an affinity for binding with calcium and is bone-seeking. Further, it is a potent enzyme inhibitor and is known to cause osteosclerosis and increased fracture rates in the osteoporotic elderly. With the approach of puberty and prior to full maturation, there occurs a spurt in skeletal growth at which time new bone formation is most active. In males, this is the time when bone fluoride accumulation is greatest. Though it may be debated whether or not fluoride is an initiator of bone cancer, it clearly appears that fluoride is a bone cancer promoter in young, maturing males. Females are less susceptible to this risk for reasons not presently known.

The response by the Public Health Service to the consistent correlation of fluoride with osteosarcoma is contrary to federal law (the Delaney amendment) and prudent policy. In other countries (e.g., Western Europe), fluoride supplementation is left to the individual; it is not put into public drinking water. If this were any other chemical agent, the Public Health Service would be calling for its removal from, rather than its intentional addition to, public water. This problem of our Public Health Service will be discussed more thoroughly in chapter 15.

When we review the various risk factors for cancer and the nutritional defenses against it, we discover that the diet for reducing our risk of cancer is the same diet recommended for general health. That is a diet composed largely of fresh vegetables, whole grains, with smaller amounts of fruit and nuts, low fat dairy products, eggs, and less protein than is now the custom. We should avoid "feed lot" meats, "jungle" fats, diary fats (a modest amount of butter is OK), sugar and refined flour, and all artificially created food. Poor nutrition is now recognized as the cause of at least 35% of our cancer. If a proper diet became a national priority, the improvement in health (and in savings of the "health" dollar) would be enormous.

The reader may have noticed that I have listed the various cancers in the chapter by their anatomical site of origin. This is standard nomenclature. But it raises the question of whether different cancers are unique or do they involve common etiologic pathways? At the present time I believe that despite their different appearances and sites of origin, most cancers have many common factors and their perceived differences are merely a sign of our present lack of understanding the cancer problem.

It is time to summarize what is known or reliably inferred of environmental factors for cancer. The following is a list of nutritional and environmental cancer factors.

Agents of defense	Risk factors
High fiber diet with whole grain cereals (wheat, rye, etc.) legumes (peas and beans) tubers (potatoes, carrots, etc.)	Fiber-deficient foods, red meat, refined flour, pastries, & sugar
	Canned foods
High vit. A foods, e.g., yellow and dark green vegetables	Deep fat fried food
	Homogenized milk and fat-rich cheese
Reduced protein intake	High protein meals (meat again)
Eat food fresh or lightly cooked and of a wide variety	Overcooked food
Clean air	Radiation, especially X-ray
Vit. C 1-2 grams/day	Cigarette smoke and engine exhaust
Sunshine	Solvents (benzene, carbon tetrachloride, paint thinners, etc.)
Vit. E 400 iu/day	
Selenium 50-100 mcg/day	Asbestos and vapors from plastics
Drink 6-8 glasses of good water per day	Insecticides and herbicides
	Oil refinery gas and glue vapors
Get 8 hours of good sleep	Fluoridated water
Maintain a positive outlook	Excess sunlight exposure (skin cancer)
	Fatigue, depression, loneliness

SELF QUIZ

1. The incidence of cancer is decreasing in the U.S. True or False?

2. Which of the following is not a protector against cancer? Vit. C, vit. E, vit. A, food fiber, 5-6 oz of protein/day, legumes. Circle one.

3. According to American Cancer Society, what percentage of cancer is due to diet? 10% 20% 30% 40% 50% Circle one.

4. In U.S. cancer research, the proportion budgeted for research in prevention of cancer is estimated to be 5% 15% 25% 35% Circle one.

5. Mammograms find breast cancer earlier than by palpation. True or False?

6. This difference, if any, makes a difference in outcome. True or False?

7. When tested in rats, fluoride increases the incidence of osteosarcoma in males but not in females. True or False?

8. Dietary fat increases the risk of breast cancer. True or False?

9. Meat eating increases the risk of colon cancer. True or False?

10. Excluding leukemia and Hodgkin's lymphoma, modern cancer treatment has significantly decreased cancer death rates. True or False?

Answers can be found on page 194.

OSTEOPOROSIS

Just as coronary heart disease is the disease US men are most certain to develop, so is osteoporosis the disease US women are most certain to develop. Osteoporosis is the progressive loss of bone density that starts several years before menopause in most women and then accelerates during menopause (or the loss of ovaries for any reason), leading to an ever increasing risk of fracture. It is more common in women of northern European extraction, in women who smoke cigarettes, and is usually worse in underweight, rather than overweight, women. The bones of the skeleton lose mass as well as minerals. Vertebral fractures are the most common but hip fractures are the most disabling. The annual US cost of treatment for osteoporotic fractures is over $10 *billion.*

A LITTLE BONE PHYSIOLOGY

Bones are constantly being made and unmade. One type of bone cell, the osteoblast, makes new bone, and another type, the osteoclast, resorbs (i.e., dissolves away) previously-made bone. During the growth phase in youth, osteoblasts out-perform osteoclasts and our skeleton grows taller and stronger. After puberty and the arrival of sex hormones, new bone formation keeps pace with bone loss. As menopause approaches, osteoblast-mediated new bone formation slows down while osteoclasts keep going as usual. Osteoporosis has begun. In men, this onset of osteoclast dominance occurs usually much later in life when testosterone fades. The gender ratio difference in the incidence of osteoporotic fractures is four females to one male.

As the bones lose mass and mineral density, they become more subject to fracture. Many of the fractures occur early in the spinal bones (vertebra); most are microfractures and unnoticed except for an occasional backache. An unmistakable sign of this process is height loss. With osteoporosis underway, any accidental fall may result in a bone fracture, such as the radius (forearm) or hip (proximal femur). In advanced osteoporosis, the hip can fracture with the slightest misstep and thus precede the fall.

Bone is similar in structure to cartilage; both are made of collagen. Bone is stronger than cartilage however, because minerals are also incorporated into its structure. Calcium is predominant but phosphorus and magnesium are also present in good quantity, plus minute amounts of silicon, boron and other minerals. Vitamin D is necessary for absorption of calcium, as is gastric hydrochloric acid. Bones do not mineralize fully unless they are placed under some physical stress such as gravity or exercise. Thus, fish have only cartilage for a skeleton, being buoyant in water, and jellyfish have no bones at all. Astronauts in gravity-free space flights will start losing bone calcium within 24 hours.

Hormones play a role in bone growth. As women approach menopause, their progesterone production falls. Progesterone production occurs only with ovulation. In many women, monthly ovulation tends not to occur in the 5-8 years prior to actual menopause. Thus, they approach menopause with progesterone deficiency and osteoporosis already underway. With menopause, estrogen production subsides dramatically. For many years, it was thought that estrogen supplementation alone would prevent osteoporosis in women. However, it is now clear that estrogen can slow the bone resorption but cannot reverse osteoporosis: it cannot restore bone already lost. Progesterone is the hormone that stimulates osteoblast-mediated new bone formation; and estrogen has the more minor role of inhibiting osteoclast-mediated bone resorption.

The decline in progesterone prior to menopause causes osteoporosis by lack of new bone formation despite normal estrogen levels. With menopause, estrogen production decreases and this allows increased osteoclast-mediated bone resorption. However, this accelerated rate of bone resorption commonly returns to its previous normal rate after 3-5 years.

Furthermore, recent research has shown that, in women athletes, strenuous exercise causes anovulatory cycles (i.e., without ovulation) and the consequent loss of progesterone; under these circumstances osteoporosis occurs despite normal estrogen levels and regular menstrual periods. Thus, it seems clear that progesterone is necessary for healthy bones in women. In women with hot flashes or vaginal dryness, estrogen may be supplemented and this would add to the success of one's osteoporosis treatment. In males, testostcronc continues until later in life. The extra testosterone helps keep their bones strong until late in life.

OTHER FACTORS IN OSTEOPOROSIS

As in other degenerative illnesses, diet is important. Daily calcium intake should be 600-800 mg, not difficult to reach by diet alone. A cup of milk or of spinach, for example, each contain about 300 mg. After age 45 or so, we become lactase deficient and do not digest milk well, developing what is called lactose intolerance, a condition that leads to flatulence and indigestion. A better alternative is a diet rich in whole grains like brown rice, millet, buckwheat, whole wheat, triticale, quinoa, and rye, as well as legumes and leafy vegetables. As noted above, a cup of leafy vegetables contains just as much calcium as a cup of milk. Cows, after all, get the calcium they need for their bones and the calcium in their milk from the pasture grass they eat. We can do the same, using other plants.

Also, whole grains and legumes are rich in magnesium. Magnesium is essential for the body and especially in regard to its important role in bone building: it helps bone incorporate calcium. Low magnesium contributes not only to osteoporosis but also increases the risk of calcification in and around joints. Magnesium/ calcium balance is the key. Milk is relatively deficient in magnesium. If milk products are included in one's diet, use only small servings of cottage cheese (the calcium-rich protein curd without either milk fats or lactose) or the fermented milk products such as yogurt or buttermilk. Calcium absorption requires vitamin D and gastric hydrochloric acid (HCl) which may need to be supplemented in those over 70. Further, the collagen portion of bone requires vitamins A and C for proper development and strength.

Almost all animals make vitamin C. A standard throughout the animal kingdom is a daily synthesis of 3-4 grams per 150 lbs of animal. We do not synthesize vitamin C and our daily dietary intake rarely exceeds 60 mg/day. For optimal bones (and health), an intake of 2 grams/day of vitamin C would seem advisable. During times of stress from other illness or recovery from fracture, vitamin C intake is especially important.

High phosphate foods tend to increase bone loss of calcium. Such foods are artificially carbonated beverages and red meats. If sufficient calcium is taken with them, the calcium-losing effect of phosphorus on bones is blunted. Under general circumstances, it is wise to avoid all artificially carbonated beverages and to restrict dietary red meat to small portions.

Meat and other sources of protein intake can have an additional negative effect on bones. When taken in amounts exceeding bodily need, the urinary excretion of their waste products (uric acid and ammonia) causes a negative calcium balance; i.e., the excretion of calcium exceeds intake. Blood tests do not reveal this urinary loss of calcium since our homeostatic mechanisms (parathyroid hormone) correct this serum deficiency by dissolving calcium from our bones to replace the loss. Osteoporosis is the result. Negative calcium balance routinely occurs with protein intake comparable to the standard American diet. This may indeed be a major cause of the increased rate of osteoporosis we see today. The previous recommendation for a protein intake of 5-6 oz. per day is excessive for adults; the correct amount is only 1.5-2 oz. daily. See Tables 1-3 .

It is interesting to compare the incidence of hip fracture in US with other countries around the world. See table 1.

Table 1. Age and sex-adjusted hip fracture rate in various areas

Area	Incidence (per 100,000 persons)
United States	98.0
Sweden (Malmo)	69.6
Israel (Jerusalem)	59.1
Finland	44.0
U.K. (Dundee, Oxford)	42.8
Hong Kong	31.5
Singapore	20.3
South Africa (black townships)	5.6

As you can see, US leads the world in hip fractures. One explanation is our high-protein diet. When calcium balance is measured in subjects eating either high protein (145 grams/day) or moderate protein (50 grams/day) diets, a negative calcium balance is found in all those eating the high protein diet, regardless of total daily calcium intake (range: 500-1400 mg/day). See table 2 below.

Table 2. Study results on calcium balance in young men on low- and high-protein diets.

No. of subjects	Calcium intake (mg/day)	Calcium balance (50 protein g/day)	Calcium balance (145 protein g/day)
9	500	+ 31	- 120
8	500	+ 24	- 116
9	800	+ 12	- 85
6	1,400	+ 10	- 84
33	1,400	+ 20	- 65

Such results suggest that vegetarians (moderate protein intake) would have better bones than omnivores, i.e., people who also eat meat and have a higher daily protein intake. This, it turns out, is indeed the case, as table 3 shows.

Table 3. Measurements of bone density in vegetarians compared to omnivores

Age groups	Density of proximal phalanx of third finger		Density of third metacarpal	
	Vegetarians	Omnivores	Vegetarians	Omnivores
50-59	1.50	1.02	1.14	0.71
60-69	1.27	0.88	1.01	0.68
70-79	1.32	0.73	1.03	0.55

All data from Family Practice Recertification Journal, vol.12, no.12, December 1990

Notice that the difference between vegetarians and omnivores increases with age. As bone density falls, fracture risk increases.

This should not be interpreted to mean that protein should be avoided. Bones need protein but *excessive* intake, as in the typical American diet, should be avoided.

The acid/alkaline balance in the body is extremely important to bones. This is determined in large part by diet. When food is metabolized, acid and alkaline products are made. If the process causes higher acidity than normal, bones lose calcium, as seen above in regard to protein intake. However, the problem is a bit more complicated than that. There are differences among peoples' metabolic processes, and, thus, their tendency to metabolic acidosis. It is important to look for metabolic acidosis in patients with osteoporosis. This can be done by saliva, urine, or blood tests. If even the slightest excess acidity is found, dietary changes can usually restore normal balance. A vegetarian diet is usually considered to be alkalizing but this is not always the case. Finding the correct diet may require trial and error testing of food changes. Though cumbersome, it is important.

The list of factors that contribute to good bones is quite extensive. It includes boron, silicon, vitamin K, vitamin B6, and probably many others yet unknown. In general, a diet of fresh unprocessed plant foods is a good bet to provide these other factors.

Exercise is essential for good bone growth. Almost any sort of exercise will do, even simple walking or swimming. The greater the exercise, the better the effect, however. Weight lifting, it turns out, or exercise against resistance is especially good for bones.

MEASURING BONE MINERAL DENSITY

Prior to the 1980s, physicians lacked an accurate test of bone mineral density (BMD). Routine X-ray, for example, can not reliably measure bone mass loss (or gain) until the change exceeds 30%. Fortunately, medical practice now has access to newer techniques that are reliable and accurate. The advent of these techniques has greatly altered the course of osteoporosis research. One such technique is photon absorptiometry, which measures the decrease of energy in a photon beam passing through tissue. Photons pass readily through skin and fat but are deflected or absorbed by the minerals in the path of the beam, in this case, bone. Single beam photon absorptiometry is good for extremity bones such as in the forearm. A modification called dual photon absorptiometry, using photons of different absorption spectra, is excellent (96-98% accurate) for bones surrounded by more body tissue such as the hip and lumbar bones. The second technique uses dual energy X-ray absorptiometry and is called DEXA. It, too, is 96-98% accurate. The third technique is a modification of CT scans and is referred to as quantified CT, or QCT. It likewise is very accurate but involves the use of much more X-ray and is more expensive. One can predict that other techniques of accurately measuring BMD will ultimately be developed because of the importance of (1) identifying patients for treatment and (2) following the course of the treatment results.

In this regard, a good home technique for identifying osteoporosis is the accurate measurement of body height. If height is being lost, the most likely cause is osteoporosis. It would be good if doctors would also do this for their patients.

TREATMENT OF OSTEOPOROSIS

As indicated by the discussion above, treatment of osteoporosis requires the proper diet, attention to a few nutritional supplements, and supplementation of the proper hormones. A question still being debated by contemporary medicine concerns the hormones. Estrogen will retard bone loss but increases the risk of water retention, fat gain, depression, loss of libido, endometrial cancer, and, most probably, also breast cancer. Contemporary medicine adds the synthetic progestins for the protection against estrogen-induced endometrial cancer but the synthetic progestins add another spectrum of possible side effects. There is a better way.

Since 1980, I have been recommending the use of transdermal natural progesterone in the treatment of osteoporosis. Natural progesterone has no known side effects, stimulates new bone formation, protects against both endometrial and breast cancer, and is well absorbed transdermally, i.e., as a cream applied to the skin. As described above, estrogen may be added, if no contraindication exists, to women with hot flashes and/or vaginal dryness. It aids in the treatment of osteoporosis by retarding osteoclast-mediated bone resorption (bone mineral loss). With or without supplemental estrogen, substantial _increases_ in BMD are regularly found by serial testing. Over a wide range of different initial BMD findings, the mean three-year improvement of BMD was >15%, compared to the expected three-year loss of 4.5%. Patients with the lowest BMD often showed the greatest improvement (25-45%). Interestingly, natural progesterone can be derived from a large number of plant sources; in this case, Mexican wild yam or soybean. No other treatment has ever provided such dramatic improvement in post-menopausal osteoporosis. Furthermore, the treatment is remarkably safe.

Despite this evidence of the remarkable improvement that can be expected from natural progesterone, research by contemporary medicine has almost totally ignored it. There are several reasons for this. One is that medical research today is generally funded by research grants proffered by the pharmaceutical industry. Since natural progesterone can not be patented, there is little prospect of profit for the industry. Thus, they have little interest in investing millions of dollars such research requires these days. Another possible reason for avoiding natural progesterone is the prevailing confusion between it and the various synthetic progestins presently available. Progestins, as a group, are fraught with undesirable side effects. Unfortunately, they have been successfully advertised to physicians as being equivalent to natural progesterone. Thirdly, most mainstream physicians are undoubtedly reluctant to be perceived by their colleagues as flirting with alternative medicine. This, however, may be changing.

The following chart depicts the percent change in bone mineral density in 63 menopausal patients using transdermal natural progesterone cream over a three-year period.

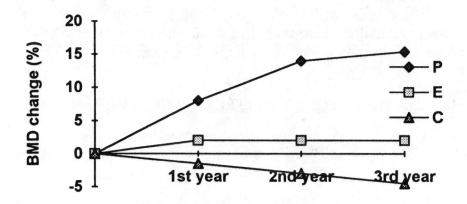

Typical lumbar BMD changes with progesterone (P), estrogen only (E), or control (C)

In this graph, it can be seen that the untreated postmenopausal patient with osteoporosis will lose 1.5% bone mass per year; that estrogen supplementation will tend to maintain bone mass: but only the addition of progesterone will increase bone mass, thus reversing the osteoporotic process.

The course of many of these patients has now been followed for over ten years while they continue to use transdermal natural progesterone. Many are now in their late 80s. Subsequent serial BMD tests show that they are maintaining their bone improvement and are escaping the fate of many of their contemporaries who have suffered hip and other fractures. Hip fractures are particularly disabling and the prospect of confinement in a nursing home is not pleasant to contemplate. Further, another unexpected dividend of natural progesterone is protection against endometrial (uterine) and breast cancer, improved general health and vitality, and an apparent retarding of aging in general.

Given the preceding discussion, it is not difficult to construct a model osteoporosis treatment program to take to your doctor in the hope that he will assist you in following it. All it requires is attention to diet, a few advisable mineral and vitamin supplements, a little exercise and natural progesterone. The addition of estrogen is a matter to discuss with one's physician but it should be known that many women do not require estrogen supplements. Hot flashes and/ or vaginal dryness are often indicators that low-dose estrogen may be helpful.

SUGGESTED OSTEOPOROSIS TREATMENT PROGRAM

Diet	Leafy green vegetables emphasized. Avoid all "sodas" and limit red meat to 3 or fewer times/week. Limit alcohol use.
Vitamin D	350-400 i.u. daily.
Vitamin C	2 gms (2,000 mg) daily in divided doses.
Vitamin A	yellow (e.g., carrots, yams, beans) and green vegetables.
Calcium	800-1000 mg/day by diet plus supplement if needed.
Magnesium	300 mg/day supplement
Zinc	15-30 mg/day supplement

Progesterone	3% cream, applied at bedtime for 24-25 days/month if postmenopausal. If premenopausal, use the cream from day 12-26 of the menstrual cycle. Use 15-20 mg/day of cream (or about one-third of a 2-oz jar or tube per month).
Estrogen	Contraindicated in diabetes, obesity, history of vascular disorders, breast cancer, endometrial cancer, or cigarette smoking. Use the least dose necessary for hot flashes or vaginal dryness, 3 weeks/month. Often not needed.
Exercise	20 minutes daily or at least 1/2 hour 3 times per week.

No cigarettes.

Report **any** occurrence of vaginal bleeding to your physician.

In applying the progesterone cream, it is advisable to choose skin areas that are rich in capillaries, such as the face and neck, the upper chest, breasts, and palms of hands, and the inside aspect of the forearms. These are all places where people blush and, therefore, with more capillaries closer to the surface of the skin for maximum absorption.

SELF QUIZ

1. Fat women tend to have better bones than skinny women do. True or False?

2. Bone can be thought of as mineralized cartilage. The chief mineral in bone is _____.

3. The bone cell that forms new bone is the

   _____.

4. The hormone that activates this bone cell in women is

   _____ .

5. The hormone that activates this bone cell in men is

   _____.

6. The hormone that doctors conventionally give women to treat osteoporosis is _____.

7. Unopposed estrogen has many possible side effects, including cancer of the uterus. True or False?

8. Exercise is good for bone building. True or False?

9. High protein diets are good for bone building. True or False?

10. The percentage of body calcium that is found in bones is 98-99%. True or False?

Answers can be found on page 194.

CHAPTER THIRTEEN
DEGENERATIVE DISEASES

Degenerative diseases are those diseases that seem to come with age and are often thought of as due to chronic "wear and tear" of one body system or another, such as arthritis, diabetes, cardiovascular disease, & cataracts. Many assume the cause is simple aging. However, the body has great resources for repair (if given the chance) and it is now becoming more clear that, like osteoporosis as discussed in the previous chapter, the deterioration observed is more likely a function of preventable impairment of repair mechanisms and not merely a function of age, per se. Chronic fluoride exposure, as example, damages the repair mechanisms and contributes to more rapid aging, as described so well by Dr. John Yiamouyiannis in his book, *Fluoride: The Aging Factor.*

THE PROBLEM OF "FREE RADICAL" OXIDATION REACTIONS

Of chief present interest is the toxicity of oxidation reactions at the cellular level caused by "free radical" formation. The term "free radical" refers to molecules with unbalanced electrons. Molecules are made of atoms in such a way that the sharing of their electrons is the force that holds the molecule together. When molecules are properly constituted, there are no electron rings that are deficient in or with excess electrons. However, molecules can suffer damage by radiation, viruses, toxic chemicals such as carbon monoxide, or from other molecules that have been damaged themselves and no longer have this perfect balance of their electron rings. They will aggressively steal a segment of another molecule to satisfy their electron requirements and thus initiate a cascade of molecular damage within the body. Such reactions may weaken a portion of a cell membrane, for example, or impair the function of an enzyme, or interrupt a repair process.

The most common site on a molecule of this "free radical" formation is an exposed oxygen atom. Oxygen is most commonly found in association with a hydrogen atom, as in water, H-OH. Radiation or some toxin may literally knock off the hydrogen; this makes the remaining portion a "free radical." Or possibly an extra electron will become added to the electron rings shared by oxygen and hydrogen thus increasing the likelihood that another oxygen will join to create a "super-oxide" molecule. Such molecules are notoriously destructive to other molecules.

Fortunately, our bodies have defenses against "free radical" danger; they function by being able to pick up or add an electron to restore balance to the affected molecule and thus neutralize the damage. These defenses, in turn, depend on a proper supply of special nutrients to maintain this important function. We now know the identity of some these special nutrients. They are vitamin C, vitamin E, vitamin A, and the mineral selenium. They are collectively termed "antioxidants" in reference to their ability to neutralize "superoxides." The process goes on continually but, under some conditions such as excess radiation, viral attacks, or autoimmune disorders, the scale of the battle rises greatly.

The molecular explanation described above may be difficult for most to grasp without a college course in biochemistry. The effect of these actions is quite commonplace, however. You may have noticed the change in smell of a vegetable oil when it becomes rancid, i.e., spoiled. That is an oxidation reaction. Butter used to become rancid when left out at room temperature; these days, however, it is protected by the addition of vitamins C and E. Iron rust is the result of an oxidation reaction. When pears or apples are prepared for canning, they sometimes turn brown when exposed to the air a bit too long. This, too, is an oxidation reaction and can be prevented by the addition of a little vitamin C. In atherosclerosis, the LDL cholesterol is now known to undergo such an oxidation reaction; this is the likely cause of plaque formation within our arteries. This explains why persons with higher intakes of vitamins C and E suffer less vascular damage. A recent study of vitamin E as a preventative for fibrocystic breast disease found, quite by accident, that eye cataract formation in those receiving vitamin E supplements was reduced by 50%. When a group of persons are accidentally exposed to, say, an herbicide, the potential toxic results are minimized in those lucky enough to have been taking extra antioxidant supplements.

Some fats (i.e., fatty acids) are more prone to oxidation reactions than others. Human breast milk has the best types of fatty acids, i.e., less subject to oxidation reactions. Cows' milk fatty acids are not quite the same. When infants were found to develop anemia after being fed for 3-4 months with cows' milk formula, the anemia was originally thought to be due to a lack of iron. When iron was added to the formula, the anemia showed up even earlier. Red blood cells have a limited life span - usually only 100-120 days. Thus they must be continually replaced by bone marrow erythropoiesis using available dietary elements. By the third month of life, all of the infant's RBCs are those made since birth. RBC membrane is made, in part, of fatty acids. Further study found that, in the case of the anemic, formula-fed infant the red blood cell membrane, instead of lasting the usual 100-120 days, was lasting only 70-80 days, thus producing the anemia. The cells' membranes were deteriorating earlier than normal as oxygen was passing into and out of the red blood cell, as is the function of red blood cells. To prevent this oxidation reaction breakdown of RBC membranes, vitamin E was given to the infants and the anemia was prevented. When this was published in medical journals, the summary (which, often, is only what doctors read) referred to the anemia as a "vitamin E deficiency anemia" instead of the true cause, i.e., the difference in the fatty acids of cows' milk compared to human breast milk. The same fats in cows' milk may be the cause of humans developing early atherosclerosis. The cows' own children, as adults, do not drink their mothers' milk.

The Fiber Factor
As described earlier in chapter 5, food fiber is important to health and the lack of fiber in our diet is strongly correlated with the development of a host of so-called degenerative diseases. That discussion will be only briefly summarized here.

In less industrialized countries, the diet is rich with fiber; i.e., from cereal grains, legumes, and tubers. In industrialized countries such as ours, these foods are less used; grain is milled (removing the fiber) and we have substituted hamburgers, French fries, cola drinks, fruit and salad vegetables which lack the fiber we need. This difference appears to largely explain the prevalence of many illnesses that are rare in non-industrialized areas. These illnesses include the following: diabetes, constipation, diverticulitis, colon cancer, heart disease and other atherosclerotic ills, obesity, hiatal hernia, gall bladder disease and gallstones, appendicitis, hemorrhoids, varicose veins, and even breast cancer.

The benefits of this type of fiber are many.

- Fiber adds bulk and retains water in our stools for easier, more prompt passage, thus reducing straining and decreasing intra-abdominal pressure which is a major factor in the development of hemorrhoids, varicose veins, and hiatal hernia.

- Fiber alters the bacteria in the intestine for better digestion and reduces the conversion of primary into secondary bile acids, which are potential cancer promoters.

- Fiber absorbs more bile acids and dilutes them within a larger stool mass and thus protects against colon cancer. With fiber, the bile itself is more soluble and less likely to form gallstones.

- Fiber reduces one's fat absorption and lowers cholesterol levels, thus reducing coronary heart disease. The fiber in grains is especially healthful; yet, with all the information printed on bread wrappers, it is difficult to find a supermarket bread containing its full complement of fiber.

It is difficult to imagine a more cost-effective way of reducing degenerative disease in our society than to return to a proper high fiber diet. No research of the treatment of these disorders will reduce their incidence or remove the morbidity they cause; the answer surely lies in the prevention of these illnesses through a sensible return to a proper diet. If enough people demand these foods, our business agriculture will provide them.

ALZHEIMER'S DISEASE (PREMATURE SENILITY)

This disease, characterized by progressive memory loss, confusion, and dementia has risen in the last twenty years from relative obscurity to virtual epidemic proportions in the US today. At autopsy, it is found associated with loss of cells from the cerebral cortex, hippocampus, and subcortical structures as well as neuritic or senile plaques (amyloid cores within nerve cells) and neruofibrillary tangles. Biochemically, there is a marked reduction in the enzyme, choline acetyl-transferase), as well as other neurotransmitters. The cause is presently unknown but environmental causes, probably multi-factorial, are suspected, including our highly processed nutrition-poor diet. Several other such possible (and preventable) suspect factors are the following:

I. The Aluminum factor

Aluminum is a known neurotoxin. Higher aluminum concentrations are usually found in the brain cells of Alzheimer's victims than in normal people of the same age. Alzheimer's disease is found more frequently in communities with higher aluminum levels in drinking water. But some argue that normal, healthy brain cells have membranes that effectively prevent aluminum from entering the cells and that it may be found there only if the cells are sick or dying from something else. Recent research, however, finds that this protection against cellular absorption of aluminum decays when fluoride is also present. Thus, exposure to fluoride <u>and</u> aluminum may be a major factor in the rising epidemic of Alzheimer's disease. Our chief source of fluoride is fluoridated water and our chief sources of aluminum are the aluminum-rich antacids and the aluminum desiccants in baking powder. Further research is needed, obviously.

II. The Aspartame and MSG factors

There is a curious Alzheimer's connection to both aspartame (an artificial sweetener) and monosodium glutamate (MSG), used as a "flavor enhancer." Both of these substances contain amino acids which, as previously discussed, are the building blocks for protein compounds such as enzymes and the neurotransmitters of the nervous system. Aspartame (trade name NutraSweet®) is a compound of aspartic acid, phenylalanine, and a methyl ester. MSG is a sodium salt of glutamic acid that occurs in food and other substances as a consequence of manufacture. Both aspartic acid and glutamic acid are "non-essential" in the sense that they can be created endogenously (i.e., within the body); however, their presence is essential for numerous intracellular metabolic functions. Furthermore, aspartic acid and glutamic acid are analogues of each other, i.e., they have almost identical chemical structures. Both are potentially neurotoxic at abnormal intracellular concentrations and, in laboratory animals, both amino acids have been found to load on the same receptors and cause the same damage to brain cells.

Phenylalanine's usual source is from food: when consumed, phenylalanine is normally converted to tyrosine. About one in 10,000 people lack, to some significant degree, the enzyme for this conversion. If phenylalanine accumulates, due to impaired conversion to tyrosine, it can lead to mental retardation and schizoid changes in children. The sign of excess phenylalanine is the excretion of phenylketone in the urine, i.e., phenylketonuria (PKU). Many states in the US have made PKU testing of the newborn mandatory since the only treatment for this condition is a low-phenylalanine diet. There may exist a partial deficiency in the converting enzyme and thus a larger number of people are at risk of some danger from high doses of phenylalanine. The use of aspartame has risen greatly in the past two decades and is found in foods where it is not expected, such as cereals, soft drinks, chewing gum and candy, and many processed foods. When ingested as a food additive, the intake of phenylalanine is greater than would occur from eating natural foods, leading to increased risk of neurologic problems.

Aspartic acid, as mentioned above, is an analogue of glutamic acid. These amino acids are neuroactive with a wide variety of actions in the brain, both as an excitatory neurotransmitter and as the precursor of GABA (gamma-amino-butyric-acid), the major brain inhibitory neurotransmitter. As reported by H. J. Roberts, MD, ingestion of aspartic acid (such as in aspartame and MSG) can cause intracellular concentrations far in excess of usual dietary sources. Brain cell function is a complex and delicate balance of neuro-transmitter activity. The disequilibrium that can potentially result from ingestion of these pure amino acids from aspartame and MSG can lead to a confusing and contradictory variety of symptoms. It is of great interest that a listing of symptoms caused by aspartame or by MSG in sensitive individuals is essentially the same list; and the symptoms occur with the same relative frequency. This is particularly important, as will be seen below.

MSG is synthetically produced by the hydrolysis of waste proteins from the dairy (whey) and meat (blood, hooves, tails, etc) industries, and from a variety of other sources. In the past twenty years, MSG sales have increased dramatically and MSG is now a multi-billion dollar industry. Despite the many reports of MSG reactions in sensitive individuals, the industry's scientific board (the International Glutamate Technical Committee, or IGTC) continues to deny their relevance. The question to be asked is - how does one prove that the onset of a headache, or memory loss, or defect in mentation, or a sudden sweat or fainting spell, or even a brain tumor is caused by MSG intake? Industry people say that the answer should be sought by large-scale double blind testing using the active ingredient (MSG) and a control placebo (containing inactive ingredients). When this was done, a large number of reactions were seen in both groups and therefore interpreted as not being due to MSG. The results were supplied to regulatory agencies such as the Food and Drug Administration (FDA) who then provided assurances of MSG safety. What was not known until recently is that, since 1978, the so-called placebo (obtained from IGTC) used in these trials was laced with aspartame which, as described above, contains aspartic acid, an analogue of glutamic acid, and the FDA has been aware of this duplicity since 1991. Since aspartic acid and MSG will cause the same reactions in sensitive people, the tests that pretended to show MSG's safety were meaningless.

The hidden sources of MSG: the following are food label descriptors that are always or often associated with the presence of MSG in food products.

These ALWAYS contain MSG:		
Monosodium glutamate	Yeast extract	Maltodextrin
Hydrolyzed protein	Yeast nutrient	Textured protein
Sodium caseinate	Autolyzed yeast	Calcium caseinate
Hydrolyzed oat flour	Yeast food	
These OFTEN contain MSG:		
Malt extract	Broth	Flavoring(s)
Malt flavoring	Stock	Natural flavoring(s)
Barley malt	Bouillon	Natural beef flavoring
"Seasonings"	Natural chicken or pork flavoring	
These CREATE MSG:		
Protease enzymes	Protease	Fungal protease

For a person with sensitivity to these ingredients, the problem of avoiding them is enormous. Under current and pending regulations, the food industry is not required to list MSG as such in food labeling unless it is added to the foods in its pure form: that is, the items above which do (or may) contain MSG in its less than pure form can be listed without identifying their MSG component. The debate over these food additives is not yet over and we are indebted to the citizens (many of whom suffer from these sensitivities) and scientists who are exposing the misinformation emanating from industry sources. One of these leaders is Mr. Jack Samuels of Northfield, IL, who supplied some of the food labeling and other information included above.

ARTHRITIC DISORDERS

Arthritis refers to stiffness, pain, and sometimes swelling and other deformities of the joints. The longer one lives, the more likely one will develop arthritis. The etiology of arthritis is unknown and several factors may be involved. These factors may include excessive wear and tear on joint surfaces, auto-immune disorders affecting cartilage or synovial tissue, viral or other infective agents in joints, and, of course, nutritional factors.

Arthritis is often divided into osteoarthritis and rheumatoid arthritis. Osteoarthritis generally causes morning stiffness and joint aching which tends to improve as the day goes on. It is less likely to cause joint deformities. Rheumatoid arthritis is more likely to cause swollen, deformed joints and its course is marked by seemingly random periods of exacerbation. It is considered to be more likely due to an autoimmune disorder in which the body's own antibodies attack joint tissue.

In either case, the healthier one's cartilage and synovial lining tissues are, the less will be the ravages of arthritis. Nutritional factors which help in this regard are vitamins C, A, B-6, & D and the minerals zinc, magnesium, and copper. Healthy, well put-together collagen fibers from which cartilage is synthesized, are dependent on sufficient vitamin C, for example, for their synthesis and repair. People with hemochromatosis (a genetic disorder in which iron absorption is excessive), commonly suffer from arthritis. In this case, the excess iron replaces other metallic ions such as the above on which the full activity of certain repair enzymes are dependent.

In 1991, a study of persons afflicted with rheumatoid arthritis demonstrated the value in this disease of a good diet. Contemporary medical treatments of rheumatoid arthritis include non-steroidal anti-inflammatory drugs (e.g., NSAIDs such as Naprosyn, ibuprofen, and others), other analgesics, cortisone, gold injections, etc. The most commonly used are the NSAIDs, all of which carry a worrisome load of adverse side effects such as gastric inflammation and ulcer. In this study, the dieter group was given a 7-10 day liquid fast (herbal tea, vegetable broth, garlic, and juice extracts from carrots, beets, celery and potatoes) followed by a diet which avoided dairy products, red meat, fish, eggs, refined sugar, citrus fruit and gluten. The control group ate their regular diet; and both groups were allowed to continue their regular medications. After the first month, the dieting group showed significant improvement in pain, morning stiffness, and in the number of tender and swollen joints. The benefits of the vegetarian diet became more obvious as the year-long study progressed; the control group showed no improvement.

Interestingly, an editorial by the American College of Rheumatology cautioned that, though the results were rather remarkable, no one should follow such a vegetarian diet without close supervision by his/her physician. In the US, studies such as these have not made a dent in the conventional treatment of rheumatoid arthritis.

Gouty arthritis is caused by joint accumulation of uric acid crystals, a waste product of protein metabolism, the urinary excretion which is reduced in the genetic disorder of gout. Persons with gout have a special reason to restrict their protein intake and to maintain adequate hydration for a good urinary output.

Other bodily aches and pains

At some time or another, everyone has bodily aches and pains, some more than others. Indeed, on occasion they can be disabling. Not arthritis, they stem from musculoskeletal connective tissue; they are given a variety of diagnostic labels – fibrositis, myofascitis, tendonitis, capsulitis, muscle strain, bursitis, soft tissue rheumatism, periarticulitis, carpal tunnel syndrome, repetitive strain injury (RSI), and many others. They occur in truck drivers, athletes, housewives, typists, beauticians, and computer operators. We are told they originate from muscle strain, bad posture, stress, depression, and even from hysteria. Perhaps in many cases, these factors do play a part. What is missing in conventional medical understanding is an appreciation of proper synthesis and repair of connective tissue. We have, these days, connective tissue (collagen fibers) that is poorly made and lacks proper repair capability. We reach maturity with collagen that is easily strained and repairs poorly. Work related strains leading to disability are threatening to bankrupt our Workers' Compensation Insurance industry.

Collagen is a non-cellular protein, which is the primary supportive material of skin, tendon, bone, cartilage and all connective tissue. It is produced by collagenoblasts (which arise from fibroblasts) in the form of smooth, strong microscopic fibers. Its proper formation requires vitamin C, vitamin A, vitamin B-6, zinc, and magnesium in addition to the protein substrate. When injured or torn, fibroblasts move in to repair it; its rate of healing is similar to bone. It is what holds all parts of our body together. When animals are slaughtered, the skin, white connective tissue, and bones are harvested, hydrolyzed, and sold to us as gelatin and hydrolyzed protein.

If proper nutrients are lacking, or in the presence of factors toxic to collagen synthesis (e.g., fluoride), our connective tissue is more easily strained or torn and its repair is weak and imperfect. The classic example of this is scurvy, caused by vitamin C deficiency. In comparing vitamin C serum levels in humans and other mammals, we find humans are deficient unless our daily intake is in the range of 1-2 grams/day. The typical US adult suffers from chronic mild scurvy and his connective tissue problems show it. If collagen fibers are torn and the repair is imperfect, fibrocytes move in and around the torn section to protect and extend the repair. These fibrocytes have tiny microfiber linkages with one another (like Velcro fasteners) which function to limit over-extension of the collagen while it is healing. Neural pain fibers follow the fibrocyte network. Over-extension or strain of the affected imperfectly healed collagen fibers triggers the pain we feel.

Treatment of this condition requires a combination of factors: support for the body area involved (e.g., wrist splints for carpal tunnel syndrome); full supplementation of the nutritional factors (vit. C, A, B-6, zinc, and magnesium); avoid postural strain (change chairs if sitting at work, take frequent breaks for limbering exercises, etc): specific massage to gently separate the microfiber linkages; a specific program of exercise to restore good muscle flexibility and tone; and allow sufficient time for good healing before subjecting the tissue to heavy strain again. We are often unaware of prolonged contraction of various muscle groups until it is too late and the pain flares again. The help of a good muscle therapist is often needed.

CATARACTS

Cataracts are progressive opacities in the body of the ocular lens. They have been mentioned in medical history of over 4000 years ago. While their cause is considered unknown, there is good information that, here too, nutrition plays an important role. Observations made in a number of long term nutrition trials for other diseases have noted a serendipitous decrease in the incidence of cataracts when vitamin A and/or vitamin E were adequately supplemented. Magnesium may also play a role. Electromagnetic radiation, e.g., exposure to radar, has caused a special type of cataract affecting the posterior membrane of the lens.

PEPTIC ULCERS AND GI BLEEDING

In young and middle age, peptic ulcers are conventionally considered to be due to gastric hyperacidity, perhaps from stress. An ulcer is an open sore in the interior lining of the stomach or duodenum. If the ulcer crater penetrates deeply enough, it can erode a gastric blood vessel and cause serious hemorrhage. Conventional treatment includes medication to decrease gastric acid. In older age, gastric bleeding may occur in a different mode. When gastroenteroscopists peer down into the stomach of an older person with gastric bleeding, they commonly see not a typical ulcer but instead finds multiple small areas of petechial (from tiny capillaries) bleeding here and there throughout the stomach. Research has shown that gastric secretion of bicarbonate (as in bicarbonate of soda) is a major defense of the stomach against digestion by its own peptic juices. For reasons yet to be explained, it is common among the elderly that they secrete much less. They also secrete less hydrochloric acid. Reducing their stomach acid further seems to be ineffective treatment for this form of gastric bleeding. What is needed is an increase in bicarbonate. Several newer medications include analogs of prostaglandins E-1 and E-2 that may be effective in stimulating gastric defenses.

Aspirin products and non-steroidal anti-inflammatory drugs all must be avoided, of course. Conventional "bland" diets are not effective. Milk, for instance, may initially soothe gastric inflammation but within an hour or so of ingestion, acid rebound is common, often making the problem worse. Surprisingly, the ingestion of peppers is not irritating to the stomach; capsicum, an ingredient of peppers, actually acts to soothe inflammation. A bit of aloe in one's diet has been found to be effective, also. All food should be well masticated. Small meals taken every 3-4 hours are better for the stomach than less frequent larger meals.

DIVERTICULITIS

Diverticulosis refers to little outpockets that develop along the wall of the colon. When inflammed and tender, this is called diverticu*litis*. The muscular wall of the colon is relatively thin, compared to the stomach. It consists of longitudinal muscle fibers with intermittent bands of concentric fibers, giving the colon a somewhat pouchy appearance. With the inadequate fiber intake of the standard American diet, constipation and higher intra-colonic pressures are the rule. The higher pressure causes little herniations between the longitudinal muscle fibers; these are the outpockets of diverticulosis. When the diet brings fermentable food products (e.g. milk products) to these areas, inflammation results, causing abdominal pain, cramps, and, usually, fever. When this occurs, doctors commonly prescribe a clear liquid diet and some antibiotic. If untreated, the diverticula may perforate and serious intra-abdominal abscesses may result. Older advice that diverticulitis was caused by seeds is found to be untrue. The true cause is high intra-colonic pressures due to poor diet; i.e., deficiency in fiber and an excess of fermentable dairy and other products. It should be recalled that, after age 35 or so years, most of us do not digest lactose (milk sugar) well whereas colon bacteria do, with rancid results.

CANCER

There is no doubt that cancer incidence increases with age. That fact, however, does not mean one should do nothing to prevent cancer if one can. The protective factors most under our own control are nutrition and the avoidance of known cancer-causing agents such as cigarette smoking and other environmental pollutants. This subject is discussed in chapter 11.

DO VITAMIN/MINERAL SUPPLEMENTS HELP?

As described in chapter 8, a vitamin/mineral supplement given to an elderly population presumably in good health and eating what is regarded as a good diet led to a "significant improvement of immunocompetence" and 40% fewer episodes of infection-related illnesses over a 12-month observation period. There should be little doubt, in this era of processed foods, that vitamin and mineral supplements are beneficial. The factor of biochemical individuality is well acknowledged and obviously implies that individual requirements of nutrients will vary from person to person. However, the fact that, in the doses usually employed, vitamin and mineral supplementation impose no risk. It is far better to use slightly more of a given vitamin or mineral than to be deficient. And, certainly no one doubts it is far better to prevent an illness than to wait and attempt to treat it after it appears. (See also chapter 5.)

CONCLUSION

Many chronic debilitating diseases usually associated with aging and called "Degenerative Diseases" are not, in fact, due to age itself. More likely, they are due to (1) years of living without the proper supply of nutrients to protect against cellular damage from oxidative reactions and (2) years of life style in which we expose ourselves unnecessarily to deleterious agents and improper diet that underlie their causation. The proper diet to optimize both goals is one which drastically lowers our intake of animal fats (including dairy fats), excessive protein, and avoids sugar, refined carbohydrates, transfatty acids, and over-processed food.

Presently, the care of chronic degenerative diseases constitutes 85% of US medical costs. It is no secret that medical costs are threatening to bankrupt our country. There are really only two ways to reduce these costs: (1) provide fewer health services, or (2) reduce the amount of illness. All the various cost-reduction schemes under consideration by the many committees and agencies today are nothing more than moving the deck chairs about on the Titanic. Is it not obvious that our primary goal should be the reduction in the amount of illness? It has repeatedly been shown throughout this book that a large percentage of illness, in particular chronic degenerative disease, is preventable. Why not extend Optimal Health concepts from the individual to the nation?

SELF-QUIZ

1. Degenerative diseases (diverticulitis, arthritis, senility, etc.) are due to old age and must be expected. True or False?

2. Fiber is good for our bowels, prevents gallstones, & lowers cholesterol. The standard American diet provides enough fiber. True or False?

3. Good sources of fiber are whole grains and legumes. True or False?

4. Because a disease occurs mainly in older folks, it can be presumed to be due to old age. True or False?

5. A "free radical" is (a) an outrageous college student not yet confined in jail or (b) an outrageous molecule with unbalanced electrons. Choose one.

6. Free radicals are products of (a) normal metabolism, (b) radiation, (c) viruses, (d) toxic chemicals, or (e) all of these. Choose one.

7. The body's defense against free radicals includes at least three vitamins and one mineral. Can you name them?
_____, _____, _____, & _____.

8. Rancid milk is an example of an oxidative reaction. True or False?

9. Arthritis is not often helped by vitamin C. True or False?

10. Cataracts may be prevented or delayed by vitamin E. True or False?

Answers can be found on the page following chapter 194.

CHAPTER FOURTEEN

MORE ON HYPERACIDITY, ULCER AND OTHER GASTRO-INTESTINAL DISORDERS

Our gastro-intestinal tract is an uninterrupted tube extending from mouth to anus, approximately 25 feet long and devilishly clever. It digests an amazingly wide variety of foods for us, extracts and absorbs the proper ingredients, and expels the remainder. Its component parts, in order, are the mouth, esophagus, stomach, duodenum, jejunum, ileum, appendix, colon, rectum, and anus. Each will be briefly described to learn its function.

Mouth: Here food is masticated and thoroughly mixed with saliva, a clear, mildly acidic solution containing the enzyme ptyalin (salivary amylase), which initiates the conversion of starch into maltose and dextrose. The tongue surface contains receptors for detecting salt, sour, bitter, and sweet; it alerts the pancreas (via the brain) that sugar is about to be absorbed into the blood, thereby stimulating the release of insulin for sugar metabolism.

Esophagus: This is the 15 or so inch tube that carries the food down the neck and through the chest into the stomach. In exiting the chest it crosses the diaphragm through a hole sufficiently loose to allow an unimpeded up and down motion of the diaphragm for respiration. (This is the site of a possible future hiatal hernia.) The esophagus moves each swallowed food bolus into the stomach by rhythmic muscular contractions called peristalsis.

Stomach: A large muscular bag the size of two fists, it is lined with velvety folds of pink epithelial cells which secrete a thickish clear mucus and a variety of digestive fluids, principally hydrochloric acid. The hydrochloric acid in the central space of the stomach accelerates the digestive process initiated by ptyalin and starts the digestion of proteins making the interior of the stomach quite a fierce cauldron of digestive activity. A thick mucus layer protects the stomach cells from the acid; and, in addition, the cells deep within the stomach lining make sodium bicarbonate for further acid defense. The masticated food is converted into a thoroughly mixed slurry in 60 - 90 minutes of stomach activity before it is released through the pylorus into the duodenum.

Excessive secretion of gastric acid is mistakenly thought by many to be the cause of peptic ulcer; whereas, in fact, gastric acid secretion is no different in those with ulcer than in those without. Peptic ulcer is due to a defect in normal defenses (gastric mucus, bicarbonate secretion, vascular supply, and intrinsic prostaglandin E-1 and E-2) and the presence of an acidophilic helical-shaped bacteria, *Helicobacter pylori*, found only in gastric lining cells. When acid is neutralized by antacids, by H-2 receptor antagonists (cimetidine, famotidine, nizatidine, or ranitidine), or by direct inhibition of the gastric parietal cell (by omeprazole), the acid-loving *H. pylori* germs are inhibited and peptic ulcers heal faster than otherwise expected. If, however, the *H. pylori* germ is not eradicated, recurrence of peptic ulcer is common. Eradication of *H. pylori* is possible by a bismuth/antacid combination treatment; i.e., Pepto-Bismol plus metronidazole and amoxicillin. The route of *H. pylori* infection is not yet known but it is known that the incidence is twice as high in gastroenterologists than in others, suggesting that spread of the germ is rather casual.

Non-pharmacologic therapy includes discontinuation of aspirin, non-steroidal anti-inflammatory drugs, and tobacco use, and strict limitation of coffee products and milk. Milk was once the mainstay of ulcer therapy but it has been convincingly demonstrated that milk results in only a temporary buffering of acid and is routinely followed by an even greater acid rebound. Ingestion of aloe vera has been found to be of benefit on occasion.

<u>Duodenum</u>: This follows a C-shaped curve 10-12 inches long and surrounds the head of the pancreas. Its secretions are strongly alka-

line. Its wall is perforated by a single orifice (sphincter of Oddi) through which both bile (for the emulsification of fats) and potent pancreatic enzymes (for digestion of fats and proteins) enter the duodenum. Lacking the thick mucus for protection against hydrochloric acid, the proximal inch of the duodenum is the favored site for peptic ulcers.

Treatment of duodenal ulcer is essentially the same as that for treatment of gastric peptic ulcer. (See chapter 13.)

Jejunum and Ileum: Collectively called the small intestine, this pliable thumb-thick, 15-20 foot long section is lined with fine folds of columnar epithelium designed to complete the digestion of our food. When fully digested, nutrients are absorbed across the cells of the small intestine for transfer into the many branches of the portal vein, which carries them to the liver. The portal vein is the only vein which carries blood somewhere else than to the heart. The small intestine can be thought of as a series of chemical factories, each with its own mission in the complex process of digestion. The food is moved along by peristalsis at a rate compatible with the digestive time for each segment. Food, in essence, is chemically broken down to its essential ingredients of amino acids, fatty acids, vitamins, minerals, etc., prior to absorption into the portal vein for transfer to the liver.

Appendix: At the juncture where the ileum empties its contents into the cecum (the bulbous antrum at the beginning of the colon), there hangs the tiny appendix, no larger than your little finger. Once thought to be a vestigial organ of no importance, it is now considered to have a role in the functioning of our immune system, similar to Peyer's patches, tonsils, etc.

Colon: Starting in the lower right corner of the abdomen, the wrist-thick, large colon carries liquidy intestinal contents up the right side, turns and crosses to the left, turns again and descends to the pelvis. In the process, water is absorbed and the intestinal contents become semi-solid and readied for evacuation out the anus. The colon contains friendly bacteria (more numerous than all the cells in your body) which complete the final digestive stages, in particular the absorption of needed minerals. Diarrhea is the early expulsion of stool still watery, and results in the loss of important minerals. Constipation, on the other hand, is a delay in proper elimination resulting in too solid stools and prolonged fermentation of stool contents by colon bacteria. The role of fiber is particularly important in keeping stool transit time proper. The muscular layer of the colon wall is thin in places and subject to herniation if internal pressures rise due to difficult stool passage; these herniations are called diverticula and become the site of toxic fermentation and inflammation (diverticulitis). (See chapter 13.)

Rectum: This is the staging area for the arriving stool prior to evacuation. It allows us to defecate at intervals rather than continuously with each wave of peristalsis. If evacuation is delayed overlong, the stool becomes progressively harder and eventually impacted. We are blessed with a nerve network that lets us know when we should evacuate stool and we are wise if we pay attention to it.

Anus: The muscular sphincter that controls stool evacuation. It is an amazingly sensitive gateway allowing, on occasion, only gas to pass and, at other times, opening wide enough for rather large and firm stools to pass. It is the location of the terminal branches of the portal vein that, unlike other veins, has no check valves to control pressure or flow. Under the increased pressure resulting from straining with constipation (or giving birth), these veins will dilate into painful masses (hemorrhoids) and sometimes bleed.

Let us now look at some interesting facts about digestion and the gastro-intestinal system. Their order of presentation has no significance.

1. Most stomach gas comes from swallowed air as a consequence of eating too fast or talking while eating, and is called *aerophagia*. Slow down, chew your food well, and enjoy your meal just as your mother told you to.

2. The esophagus is so competent in its function that it is possible to stand on your head and swallow beer (or any liquid) without spilling a drop.

3. When young and under stress, the stomach might make more acid and, also, shunt blood away from the stomach to the muscles. Ulcers may result. The acid is not the real cause of ulcers. There exists a bacterium that proliferates well in a strong acid environment. It is this bacteria (described above) which is the real cause of the ulcer. Without the presence of the bacteria in your stomach, extra acid does not cause ulcers.

4. When older and under stress, the stomach cells make less sodium bicarbonate and thus can not protect itself against normal digestive action. Antacids or acid-restricting medication (e.g. Tagamet) will not correct this problem. The answer is to lower stress and keep some sodium bicarbonate on hand.

5. After age 70 or so, 50% or more of us make very little hydrochloric acid. Prior to that, we may make this acid only at mealtime. Calcium absorption requires vitamin D and hydrochloric acid. Eating properly and taking calcium supplements will do us no good if we lack gastric hydrochloric acid. Lack of hydrochloric acid also results in indigestion, which is often misinterpreted as hyperacidity and leads to prescriptions for antacids and Histamine-2 receptor antagonists. In this age group, hydrochloric acid supplements at meal time are much more likely to be beneficial than blocking hydrochloric acid.

6. Stomach digestive juices are lethal to most germs and thereby protect us from germs in the food we eat. Only a few can survive the stomach cauldron. One, *Helicobacter pylori*, grows well in a strong acid environment and can lead to ulcers. Another is the bacteria named *Vibrio*

cholerae, the agent of cholera (life-threatening diarrhea). Others, however, are beneficial such as *Lactobacillus acidophilus* which inhabits our colons and can safely make the journey through the stomach. Certain germs that live in our intestines are the source of the vitamin K we need for blood clotting. Vegetarians, it is said, get their vitamin B12 from germs that live in their gut. We evolved, after all, by eating unsterile food.

7. Milk is not meant for grownups. Lactose is the only sugar synthesized by animals (mammals, in their breasts). It is a disaccharide that requires a special enzyme (lactase) in our stomach for digestion. At birth we make plenty of the enzyme. If black, we lose that enzyme at age 17 or so; if Asian, we lose the enzyme by age 25; if our ancestors are from a Nordic area, we lose it at age 35-45. After we lose the enzyme we cannot digest lactose. It passes through us like so much sawdust and, on entering the colon, is fermented by bacteria there. This leads to gas and indigestion. Yogurt can be substituted since it is made with a culture (more germs) that digests the lactose for us. Cheese, a protein curd without lactose, is also OK.

8. High intra-abdominal pressure is a result of delayed stool transit; it can result in hiatal hernia, diverticulitis, hemorrhoids, bloating, and pain. Delayed stool transit can be corrected with sufficient water and food fiber. Our diet during millennia of evolution contained fiber-rich foods; our modern diet is fiber-deficient. We should switch to eating leafy vegetables, legumes, tubers, and whole grains. Transit time can be easily tested: eat some fresh corn and observe when the kernels are passed in a stool. A good transit time is 18 hours or so; a bad transit time is >36 hours.

9. High fiber diets also lower cholesterol, aid in preventing gallstones, and lower the risk of colon cancer and heart

disease. All these benefits are obtained just by eating whole foods and less processed foods.

10. Mechanical de-gutting of chicken results in extensive contamination of the carcass with *Campylobacter* bacteria (a common intestinal inhabitant in fowl) which, if ingested can cause diarrhea and fever. Though commonly confused with viral gastroenteritis, this infection responds to erythromycin antibiotics. This infection was much less common when processing of chickens was done by hand. After cutting up a chicken carcass in your kitchen, it is wise to thoroughly clean the counter to avoid spread of the germ to other foods placed on the counter.

11. Extensive antibiotic supplementation given to animals has resulted in the emergence of antibiotic-resistant organisms (e.g., salmonella, etc.) in the milk, eggs, and meat we eat causing serious difficult-to-treat illnesses. As this problem of antibiotic-resistance spreads, we risk losing all antibiotic benefit. This would be a medical catastrophe.

12. Given today's food supplies and environmental toxicity risks, the vitamin supplements most certain to be needed are vitamin C (1-2 grams/day), vitamin E (400-600 units/day), and betacarotene (15 mg/day).

The above list is naturally incomplete but should serve as a springboard for opening minds about the importance of paying attention to our G-I system. It's there to help us and, as a rule, is wiser than we think.

SELF QUIZ

1. Saliva contains a digestive enzyme. What is its name?

   _____

2. The esophagus passes through a hole in the diaphragm. True or False?

3. Fat digestion occurs in the stomach. True or False?

4. For ulcers, milk is a good antacid. True or False?

5. Most peptic ulcers occur in the duodenum. True or False?

6. The function of bile is to _____ fats. Fill in word

7. The pancreas, in addition to secreting insulin, excretes strong digestive enzymes directly into the duodenum. True or False?

8. Bile is made by the liver and is passed to the duodenum by the common bile duct. Along the way, an extra reservoir of bile is kept on reserve. What is its name?

   _____

9. Diverticulitis is caused by eating tomato and grape seeds. True or False?

10. The appendix has no known function. True or False?

Answers can be found on page 194

FRUSTRATING TWENTIETH CENTURY ILLNESSES

Throughout medical history, the prevailing health philosophy was one of harmony and equilibrium. Illness was seen as a disturbance or lack of harmony in life processes. Early Greek physicians taught that all matter consisted of elements and qualities in a dynamic opposition (alliance) to one another; and that balance or harmony was a necessary condition for a healthy life. Hippocrates instructed his students that both the disturbing forces (producing disharmony/illness) and the healing forces were of natural, and not supernatural, origin. The physician's goal was to restore harmony.

The 20th century has produced an aberration in the course of medical history. Even as Bernard, in mid-19th century, was teaching the concepts of heterogeneity, harmony and homeostasis, the discoveries by Pasteur and Koch of disease germs (1860s), followed by the discovery of penicillin (1930s), caused an unfortunate tilt in medical thinking away from heterogeneity and the harmony of physiological processes, and toward a single-minded emphasis on the disease vector. The theory of the "magic bullet" was born. We forget that Pasteur, on his deathbed, was reported to assert that Bernard was right - "the germ is nothing, the terrain (internal milieu) is everything." And so the world forgot that merely killing a germ does not restore health any more than does setting out poison to kill mice repair the holes in one's home. Ignored was the age-old wisdom that only the return to physiological harmony can restore the healing power of nature.

Thus it is that conventional medicine is in a terrible state of disarray. Doctors' offices are full of patients with diseases not well understood and which are being treated without much success. Pharmaceutical technology has provided full quivers of antibiotics (against which bacteria are acquiring an ever-increasing resistance) and drugs for the amelioration of symptoms; but healing and recovery is becoming ever more rare. The touted extension of life expectancy is not due to our antibiotics, immunizations, or "miracle" drugs but, instead, should be credited to better public hygiene - clean water, better food handling, sewage sanitation, and improved housing - leading to a major reduction in infant mortality, the prime statistical factor in our 20th century increase in life expectancy. Our young, however, lack the vigor and physical stamina of those a generation ago. From middle age on, the present picture is one of mysterious and progressive deterioration. The old diseases (e.g., tuberculosis, malaria) are making a comeback, other diseases (e.g., cancer) are increasing, and a host of new diseases now predominate; diseases with names such as chronic fatigue syndrome, non-Hodgkin's lymphoma, carpal tunnel syndrome and other connective tissue ills, osteoporosis, auto-immune disorders (e.g., thyroiditis, lupus, Sjogren's syndrome), mental illness and pre-senile deterioration (e.g. Alzheimer's), and viral infections never before heard of (e.g. HIV). Our treatments are expensive, symptom-oriented, and largely ineffective. Something has gone wrong with our disease resistance and our healing ability; and 20th century medicine does not know what to do about it.

It is becoming ever more clear that our immune system and general healing powers have deteriorated. What answer could there be other than poor nutrition and increased environmental toxins? This is where our research technology and our priorities should be applied. Success in health and healing lies in proper nourishment, exercise, and the avoidance of toxic agents. Wholesome food does not mean only sanitized food; it means food with a full complement of its innate nourishing ingredients and the absence of toxic chemical additives. We need food that is fresh, unprocessed, whole, and unadulterated. Our food suppliers will meet this need if we demand it. Food should be chosen not for its convenience but for its wholesomeness. In the cultural upheaval and fragmentation of modern society, we have lost age-old food wisdom (the so-called "ethnic" diets); nutritional re-education should become a national priority. Nothing, at this time in history, could be more healthful or cost effective.

In previous ages, exercise was simply a part of working and living. Today, we are paving our school playing fields to provide space for student parking; we drive to every shopping and business location; we heat our homes by turning a switch on the wall; less than 2% of our families live on working farms and, even there, manual labor has been largely replaced by mechanical devices. Our bodies thrive on exercise and they will atrophy from lack of it.

Our environment has become poisonous. We talk of the toxic effects of smog but our urban air remains fouled with petrochemical byproducts. Our once clear ground waters are all contaminated with toxic industrial waste. Mothers' breast milk carries pesticide; neurotoxic lead and aluminum are found in our brains; our bones are saturated with fluoride; our livers become the repository of food-borne insecticides and trans-fatty acids; and electromagnetic waves of unknown biotoxic consequences radiate through our bodies. Our drinking water is disinfected with chlorine (recently correlated with bladder and rectal cancer) instead of safe ultraviolet light or ozonization. We must consider applying our technology research to these concerns rather than, say, space exploration. This world, Earth, is our home; it is in our interest to keep it healthy for human life.

After a century of ignoring whole body healthfulness and the single-minded emphasis on destroying the disease vector, it is time to return to the paradigm of physiologic balance (harmony), i.e., that true healing stems from the multifactorial dynamism of internal equilibrium. Now is the time for a renaissance, an awakening of true bio-medical nutritional research. We have a choice: we can apply our technology to creating a century of better health for all, or go on as we are and suffer a century of modern incurable plagues.

Let us take a brief look at some of the frustrating 20th century illnesses.

CHRONIC FATIGUE SYNDROME

Oddly, this disease appears to strike the relatively well off and those supposedly in the prime of life. Its primary symptom is a variable, often severe, fatigue of long duration (over 3 months and frequently much longer) but is accompanied also with memory loss and inability to concentrate, sleeping disorders, muscle and joint pains, a deepening sense of despair, low grade fever, and periodic episodes of lymph gland swelling similar to a mild case of mononucleosis. Laboratory tests frequently show low leukocyte (white blood cell) counts and, sometimes, a rising titer of antibodies against fungal (e.g. *Candida albicans)* and/or viral (e.g., Epstein-Barr) agents normally considered harmless or relatively benign. Its cause has not been found. It would appear, however, that underlying the various manifestations is an impaired immune system.

When chronic fatigue syndrome first became noticeable, many patients were given such diagnoses as neurasthenia (a favorite of the 19th century), simple depression, or malingering. But CFS, with its fevers, its recurring adenopathy, and its low white blood cell counts is none of these; it is the classic 20th century illness. *Something* is impairing the immune system of people who otherwise should be enjoying good health.

No therapy by contemporary medicine cures CFS. Antibiotics, gamma globulin, anti-depression medication, psychotherapy, and group counseling have all failed these patients. In some, gradual remission and eventual recovery occurs; in others, the symptoms drag on for years without any true recovery.

Recently, a fortuitous discovery was made. Physicians in England studying patients with CFS consistently found low red blood cell magnesium levels despite normal serum levels in these patients. Magnesium, after potassium, is the second most important intracellular mineral electrolyte. Homeostatic mechanisms maintain a stable serum level of magnesium, even at the expense of lowered intra-cellular levels. When given oral supplemental magnesium, neither their cellular magnesium levels nor their symptoms improved. They were then given intramuscular injections of magnesium. When retested two weeks later, their cellular magnesium levels were back to normal <u>and</u> their CFS symptoms had cleared!

What had happened here? Certainly, simple magnesium deficiency is not the cause of CFS One likely explanation is that, whatever caused the CFS, cell membranes had lost their ability to maintain intracellular magnesium at normal levels. Once the magnesium was lost, the hundreds of enzymes for which magnesium is a co-factor also lost their ability to function adequately, the net effect of which causes the multiple symptoms of CFS - the fatigue and impaired immunocompetence, leading to the observed loss of resistance to otherwise benign viral, bacterial, and fungal invaders, with low grade fever and leukopenia. This enzyme dysfunction apparently included the enzymes driving the cell membranes' biochemical "pumps" for the selective intracellular magnesium concentration. Only by giving a "surge" of magnesium by injection could sufficient magnesium re-enter body cells. Once intracellular magnesium was restored, the cells resumed normal function and the chronic fatigue syndrome cleared.

Given that explanation of the effects, what could be its cause? The most probable etiologic hypothesis is the multitude of environmental factors previously suggested: our nutritionally deficient diet, pervasive petrochemical toxins, electromagnetic radiation (many patients are computer-users), excessive reliance on antibiotics, insecticides and herbicides, general stress, etc. These will be more extensively identified later in this chapter. CFS is just one illness among a number of others that has as its basis the broad spectrum of our unique 20th century health risks.

The description in the paragraphs above provides a suggestion for diagnosis and treatment of CFS. Lacking a specific diagnostic test, the presence of low intracellular magnesium is important. Treatment should include restoring this valuable electrolyte, either by IM or IV injection, in addition to choosing a fully nutritious diet and adopting a life style that avoids as many of the environmental risk factors as possible.

CHAPTER FIFTEEN

HIV AND AIDS

AIDS (Acquired Immune Deficiency Syndrome) is certainly the most notorious disease of the century, given its present fatality rate of near 100%. Since first recognized in the mid-1970s, and until just recently, it was thought that AIDS was caused by HIV (Human Immunodeficiency Virus) whose presence is detected by HIV antibodies. Recently, doctors are seeing AIDS patients who show no sign of HIV antibodies, suggesting that acquired immune deficiency syndrome may be caused by factors other than HIV. Also, researchers at the Pasteur Institute in Paris, where HIV was first isolated, now believe that HIV is insufficiently pathogenic to be the sole cause of AIDS; i.e., that AIDS requires, in addition, another pathogen (such as the agents that cause "viral" pneumonia or a herpes infection) or other toxic substances for HIV to become an active infection. The picture is even more confusing since the discovery that several different strains of HIV co-exist. The etiology and management of AIDS is an open question.

The major targets of HIV are white blood cells, specifically the CD4+ T-lymphocyte, macrophages and monocytes. Once HIV enters the cell, it sheds its envelope protein and converts its own RNA to a double strand of DNA which can invade the host cell's nucleus, a process known as "reverse transcription." Once inserted in the host DNA, it causes the manufacture of new viral components which become more HIV when released into extracellular fluid by a "budding" process through the host cell's membrane and thus they continue the spread of the infection.

Many infected individuals carry HIV without symptoms for a number of years as can be shown by the presence of high titers of HIV antibody and low titers of the virus in the blood. Despite these antibodies, viral replication does continue. In time, immune deficiency progresses and patients become more susceptible to mild opportunistic infections: this stage is termed ARC (AIDS related complex). It then leads into full-blown AIDS in which each secondary infection is potentially lethal.

The most critical effect of HIV is to kill the CD4+ T-lymphocytes and inactivate CD8+ cytotoxic lymphocytes. These two cells represent one of the body's primary methods of killing HIV. The loss of these cells, principally CD4 T-cells , causes immunodeficiency and ultimately the disease picture known as AIDS. Our usual immune defenses consist of humoral and cellular factors. In this case, the humoral factor (antibodies production) works fine but the cellular factors (the white blood cells that kill invaders) are themselves victims of the infection.

The creation of immunodeficiency opens the door to opportunistic infections of all sorts but principally *Pneumocystis Carinii*, toxoplasmosis, herpes, cryptosporidium, mycobacterium avium complex, hepatitis, tuberculosis and syphilis. The care of the patient requires vigilant attention to the possible presence of any or all of these and each must be treated promptly and as thoroughly as possible with appropriate medication.

Medical attempts to stop HIV replication in infected host cells have involved three drugs, AZT, ddI, and ddC, all reverse transcriptase inhibitors. Unfortunately, medical evidence that any of them slow the infection or prolong life is problematic.

It is of interest that HIV infection creates no disease, generally, in other mammals. The lack of an animal model impedes research. At this time, attempts are underway to develop genetically altered mice for this purpose. The startling emergence of this terrible disease raises several questions: is the morbidity and mortality of HIV due to mutation of new, more deadly strains of this retrovirus, or, did something happen to man's immune resistance making him/her more susceptible to the virions?

AIDS has brought several corollaries worth mentioning. These are:

1. Physicians are being confronted with a disease they cannot "fix." This is discomforting to physicians who have previously enjoyed the role of heroic rescuer of ill patients.

2. AIDS has re-introduced the deeper dimension of what it means to be a physician caring for patients they cannot heal; that is, the discovery that their real role is one who CARES for the patient, a calling over and above the mere treatment of an illness.

3. No amount of antibiotic treatment is successful without a healthy immune system. Antibiotics may kill or suppress the vast majority of the infectious organisms against which the antibiotics are considered "effective"; but *cure* of the infection requires the immune system to complete the job. Autopsy studies of AIDS victims found that *every infection supposedly treated effectively by antibiotics was still present in their body tissues!*

OTHER VIRAL AND FUNGAL INFECTIONS

The advent of antibiotics initiated an era that promised the control of infections. What was overlooked was the fact that antibiotics (usually fungi-based) are effective only against bacteria, and then only against some of them. Success in clearing one bacteria (or set of bacteria) merely creates the ecologic niche for the flourishing of other organisms; and this is exactly what happens. Yeast overgrowth is a well-recognized complication of antibiotic use. Pneumonia caused by Pneumococci, previously common in the elderly, is now replaced by more virulent antibiotic resistant strains or viral pneumonia. Acquiring infections is more than mere happenstance; it frequently is associated with a depressed immune system. Our 20th century lives are full of chemicals and other agents that depress our immune system. A broad spectrum of resistant bacteria and viruses (for which no antibiotic is effective) now are common.

CORONARY HEART DISEASE

As described in chapter 9, CHD, now our #1 killer, was a rarity in young - middle age men prior to the mid-1900s. See chapter 9 for a more complete discussion.

CANCER

As described in chapter 10, cancer incidence continues to rise, an increase not explained by life extension. Breast cancer, for instance, is occurring at younger ages and its incidence has increased from one in thirty women to one in nine as women age. Several probable factors for this deserve serious attention. One is the known increase of toxic pesticide and herbicide residue in breast fat. Dioxin, DDT, DDE, and PCB's (polychlorinated biphenyls), all with a long half-life, are found in increasing concentration in breast fat. Studies indicate, for instance, that the fat tissue of those with breast cancer has a 50-60% higher concentration of PCBs. Many of the pesticides are petroleum-based, fat soluble toxins that, when ingested by fish or animals, accumulate in their fatty tissues. These harmful toxins move up the food chain to eventually reach humans. They need not be present in food; exposure by simply breathing can be sufficient. The National Academy of Sciences has now accepted that the herbicide, Agent Orange (containing dioxin), caused the increased incidence of non-Hodgkin's lymphoma, soft-tissue sarcoma, and Hodgkin's disease in Viet Nam veterans and, possibly, birth defects in their children.

Many toxic petroleum-based chemicals permeating our environment have potent estrogenic activity. They emanate from pesticide use, from plastics we use, and from solvents such as found in the backing of modern carpets. Such agents are totally foreign to human metabolism and wreak havoc throughout the body. The toxic potency of some of them is truly astounding - creating effects at nano-gram levels (i.e., 1 *billionth* of a gram). The estrogenic activity of these silent invaders is being credited with not only the increase of breast cancer but also the decline in healthy, motile sperm now being observed in men. A well-studied example of inappropriate and toxic estrogenic compounds is diethylstilbestrol (DES), previously used sometimes in pregnant women: its influence on the female fetus is such that, later in her life, she is at increased risk of cervical cancer.

Synthetic (man-made) chemicals have become ubiquitous: over 3,000 such chemicals are intentionally added to foods, over 700 are found in drinking water, and, in the Great Lakes for example, 300 synthetic chemicals are present, including DDT, PCBs and dioxin. These 20th century chemicals are inimical to natural biochemical functions and an increased cancer risk is just one of their dirty tricks.

Radiation, particularly X-ray, can induce cancer. Not too long ago, shoe stores provided fluoroscopes for patrons to see the bones of their own feet in the shoes they were buying. Because of the later recognition of X-ray-induced breast cancer, these machines are no longer used. This breast cancer risk is sufficiently great so that medical students now are taught that bronchitis and even pneumonia in young girls should be treated without resorting to chest X-ray, if at all possible. The fact is we live in a sea of radiation - from radio and TV broadcasts, microwave radiation from TV sets, high voltage electric lines, desk computers, hair dryers and other electrical equipment held in close proximity, radar, etc., all permeating our body with potential for toxic effects, including cancer.

DISEASES OF HORMONE IMBALANCE

The latter half of the 20th century has seen a tremendous rise in diseases of hormone imbalance. Premenstrual syndrome (PMS), infertility and early miscarriage from luteal phase failure, fibrocystic breasts, irregular and heavy menstruation often leading to hysterectomy, obesity in females, and cancer of the breast, uterus, and ovary are all hormone related and typical of estrogen dominance. Males exhibit their share of hormone imbalance by falling sperm counts, increased incidence and earlier onset of prostatism and prostate cancer. While some observers attribute much of this to earlier detection, the fact remains that something has caused widespread hormone imbalance throughout the industrialized world.

The most likely cause of hormone imbalance in adults is exposure to petrochemical xenobiotics during early embryo life. The same problem occurs in multiple animal species, as detailed in the book, *Our Stolen Future,* and there is no reason to think that humans are immune to these toxic compounds. Females grow up unable to produce progesterone to balance their estrogen. Males grow up to find that they, at age

40, have only half the sperm count their fathers did. Males make considerable estradiol but its carcinogenicity is defused by their usual higher concentrations of testosterone and progesterone. When these two hormones are no longer produced in adequate quantity, relative estrogen dominance is the result. As a consequence, prostate problems (including prostate cancer) are becoming common in men before age 50.

Through the work of scientists around the world (e.g., Dr. E. Cavalieri, professor at the Eppley Institute for Research in Cancer and Allied Diseases, U of Nebraska Medical Center, and many others) we now know that estrogen is the probable cause of hormone-dependent cancers. The facts are: (1) estrogen dominance increases its carcinogenic potency; (2) estrogen dominance results from relative progesterone deficiency; and (3) progesterone deficiency is the result of dysfunctional ovaries and testes that were harmed by exposure to xenobiotics during the formative embryo stage of life.

To date, research into these matters has largely ignored the factor of relative progesterone deficiency. In fact, physicians rarely test their patients' progesterone levels. Conventional medicine continues to prescribe estrogen to women who don't need it and almost never prescribe progesterone to women who are deficient in it. They do, however, prescribe synthetic progestins that offer some protection against endometrial cancer but this does not really solve the estrogen dominance problem. Only real progesterone can do that.

This topic is far too large to discuss in any detail in this book. For those who are interested, I refer you to the several books I have authored or co-authored concerning hormone balance. They are *Natural Progesterone* (available from BLL Publishing, P.O. Box 2068, Sebastopol, CA 95473), *What Your Doctor May Not Tell You About Menopause*, and *What Your Doctor May Not Tell You About Premenopause*, both available from Warner Books. While progesterone supplementation can be of great help to people deficient in it and suffering from estrogen dominance, the real solution to the problem will come only by learning to keep our food and living environment free of toxic compounds.

DYSFUNCTIONAL CITIZENS

There is a rising concern that the mounting number of citizens euphemistically called "street people" are, in fact, not merely out of work but, in large degree, are organically dysfunctional and unable to cope with modern life. This, too, is a hallmark of the 20th century. Many factors, of course, are involved: drug use, dysfunctional homes and upbringing, malnutrition, lack of marketable skills, chronic illness, the economic times, etc. But one factor that has largely been overlooked is defective embryogenesis. As in growing a garden or raising crops or animal husbandry, the most important concern is the fertility of the ground or the healthy vitality of the parents. The most important time in the health of the expected crop or offspring occurs *prior* to the planting (i.e., the preparation of the soil) or fertilization of the ovum by the sperm. The formation of healthy ova or sperm (i.e., of gametes during meiosis) with a full complement of normal genes requires the best possible nutritional status and absence of biologic toxins. Defective ova or sperm chromosomes are indelible hazards to all subsequent growth and development.

After fertilization, the first two-three weeks of embryogenesis, when cell differentiation is first forming, are also extremely important. These few weeks of germ cell formation and early embryogenesis are critical; and they generally occur *before* the mother is aware she is pregnant.

A recent clear example of latent deleterious effects secondary to nutritional deficiency is the correlation of neural tube defects (e.g., spina bifida) in newborns to deficient folic acid (a B vitamin found in fruits, liver, legumes, and vegetables). It is now concluded that at least proper maternal diet or even supplementation with this inexpensive vitamin could eliminate half of such congenital deformities. Another example might be the fetal alcohol syndrome, i.e., mental retardation and facial deformities secondary to maternal alcohol use and malnutrition.

Given the prevailing malnutrition secondary to dietary misinformation, over-processed and nutritionally deficient foods, trans-fatty acids, and the flood of environmental toxins, it is little wonder that children are increasingly developing with damaged genetic goods. If one wishes to preview the future of a society fully impacted with such a problem, read the small chapter entitled "The Iks" in the book, *The Lives of a Cell* by Lewis Thomas (1974). The Iks are tribal nomadic hunters forced to live as farmers on poor hillside soil in northern Uganda. Dr. Thomas describes their descent into "an irreversibly disagreeable collection of unattached, brutish creatures, totally selfish and loveless" that "breed without love or even casual regard." They "defecate on each other's doorsteps" and laugh only at other's misfortune. For them, society has become unworkable. Does this not seem vaguely familiar when one observes the street people in our major cities?

How does our society respond to this dilemma? We give these people a small remittance, we process them in our emergency rooms and social welfare agencies, we move them from place to place; but we are doing nothing to stem the flowing tide, we are ignoring the source from which they emerge. Allowing, even fostering, a subclass that lives and procreates in an environment of malnutrition, toxic exposure, and social dysfunction will more surely destroy the society or nation than any outside force imaginable. This problem is larger than AIDS. We might learn something from the example of the Iks.

THE THREAT OF MEDICAL "CARE"

For the first time in medical history, doctors have access to truly potent medicines. During the 19th century, medical progress was characterized by advances in understanding pathological process, of more accurate delineation of disease, and refinements in diagnosis. The lack of effective therapy led to an atmosphere of nihilism among practitioners. The 20th century has seen an explosion of potent and truly effective medical interventions. My father's medicine bag carried urinary catheters and tourniquets, scalpel and scissors, a glass syringe or two with needles, digitalis, morphine, sedatives, calomel, nitroglycerine and aspirin. Now we have medications that would appear miraculous to him: cortisone, antibiotics, anti-hypertensives, tranquilizers, diuretics, insulin, anti-inflammatories of all kinds, and many, many others. The prospect of altering bio-logic processes with readily available drugs has never before been encountered.

From Hippocrates to the present, medicine's credo has been "primum non nocere" (above all, do no harm). In the absence of such potent drugs, this admonition was not all that difficult to follow. Now, the attraction of powerful medications (of playing God, as some prefer to call it) blurs the line for many physicians and the credo hangs around in the background in our thinking, rather than in the foreground where it still belongs. Medical treat-ments, if inappropriate or mismanaged, now constitute a real and potent threat to health. The book, *Matters of Life & Death: Risks vs Benefits of Medical Care* by Eugene D. Robin, MD, is a good in-troduction to this problem. This is the topic of the next chapter and will not be further pursued here except to indicate its place as a 20th Century health risk.

SUMMARY
In the US, the 20th century has seen a great apparent improve-ment in living conditions, food distribution, education level, rela-tive affluence, public welfare assistance, access to medical care and the nature of medical care. We have the highest doctor per capita ratio in the world. And despite all this, we have also seen a rise in many illnesses - cardiovascular disease, cancer, hypertension, im-mune disorders, musculoskeletal disorders, and the emergence of new diseases. The cost of medical care has risen dramatically (twice the rate of inflation) in the past decade and now exceeds 14% of the gross national product, far more than any other nation. Total medi-cal costs were 838 *billion* dollars in 1992, over $3000 per person,* and hit 1 *trillion* in 1994. Yet we lag in many health categories: we rank 15th in the world in infant mortality, 16th in the world in fe-male life expectancy, and 35th in the world in male life expectancy, and our children compare poorly in physical aptitude. Surgeon Gen-eral Koop estimated that 76% of our annual deaths are nutritionally related. We are world leaders in cardiovascular disease. Treatment of chronic disease accounts for 85% of the national health care bill.

Clearly, we are not doing a good job in achieving a healthy popu-lation. The fault can not be laid to the doctors; getting healthy is a matter of prevention, not of more care once illness strikes. Prevent-able illness makes up at least 70% of our medical costs and accounts for eight of the nine leading real-cause categories of death (980,000 deaths per year). Prevention is a matter of nutrition and decreasing our exposure to toxic products during all stages of life. Our national health policy should have as its core the education of our people in the creation of a new understanding of health and the prevention of illness.

*National Center of Health Statistics (DHHS publication no. [PHS] 92-1232.) *NEJM*, 29 July 1993, vol. 329, no. 5, 321-325.

SELF QUIZ

1. Great medical advances were made during the present century. True or False?

2. The US leads the world in the # of doctors per capita and money spent per capita on medical care. True or False?

3. As a result, the rate of illnesses in the US is falling. True or False?

4. Many illnesses such as heart disease, cancer, mental illness, hypertension and immune disorders increased during the present century. True or False?

5. The % of our annual deaths related to bad nutrition is estimated to be __ %.

6. AIDS (acquired immune deficiency syndrome) is always due to contagion by HIV (human immunodeficiency virus). True or False?

7. Chronic fatigue syndrome is primarily a psychological illness. True or False?

8. Congenital disorders can be due to nutritional factors. True or False?

9. "Street people," in general, are normal people who have merely lost their jobs and have no money. True or False?

10. Pesticides kill bugs in plant foods but don't hurt people. True or False?

Answers can be found on page 194.

CHAPTER SIXTEEN
IATROGENIC DISEASE

Going to the doctor these days can be risky business. In generations past, a basic tenet of medical care was "Primum non nocere" (above all, do no harm). Today, that dictum has been modified to "do as little harm as possible." Even that, as we shall see, is becoming operationally impossible. The patient now must learn to look out for himself.

Iatrogenic disease refers to health problems resulting from treatments by medical authorities. This is not a health problem of small consequence nor is it new. The history of medicine is replete with many examples, from "therapeutic" bleeding to "laudable pus." What is most curious about them is the fact that the problems created (so obvious in retrospect) were, in their time, so long unrecognized. Perhaps this is still true. More importantly, a recent study found 25% of hospital admissions to be directly related to medical mismanagement of some kind or another. It is appropriate, therefore, that we take a good look at this problem. An excellent book to read on the subject of iatrogenic disease is Dr. E. D. Robin's *Matters of Life & Death: Risks vs. Benefits of Medical Care.*

Almost all medications have undesirable side effects, which are often not fully realized by the patient or his/her doctor. The treatment of one condition may exacerbate another. This is not rare; in fact, it is generally the rule. Sometimes, an errant health notion is so widespread throughout the health community that literally millions of people suffer from it without suspecting the cause. (Dr. Robin then calls it an "iatro-epidemic") Various examples are now well known: the use of tetracycline antibiotics in childhood (caused discoloration of developing teeth); the Sippy diet for ulcers (milk causes acid rebound); the use of pHisohex baby powder (hexachlorophene is

(187)

neurotoxic); excessive dietary protein advice of 30 years ago; the excessive cola drinks of today; and the casual use of radium and X-ray just one generation ago. All of these induced iatrogenic disease in large numbers.

The doctor doesn't set out, of course, to purposefully harm the patient. But somehow he/she can't seem to help it. Let us look at some of the reasons for the problem.

1. The phenomenal ongoing proliferation of medications and treatments available make it impossible for even the most responsible doctor to keep up with the ever expanding knowledge of possible contraindications and side effects, let alone the interactions between them when used in combinations.

2. Not all side effects are known when the drug is released for general use. Animal tests and limited clinical trials are simply incapable of providing a broad enough database for reactions that might be quite rare.

3. Surprising as it may seem to some, "spin-doctoring" is rampant in medical literature. Doctors who are not impartial in their advocacy of a drug or treatment about which they are reporting often write articles published in even the most prestigious medical journals. It is very easy to exaggerate presumed treatment benefit and minimize undesirable side effects. Medical research is financed primarily by drug companies hoping to make money selling a drug. They choose researchers who will, in effect, put the right "spin" on their results. Studies that are not favorable (to the pharmaceutical company's interest) do not get published. Medical research careers often depend on satisfying the desires of the pharmaceutical interests that pay for the research. It is important to remember that pharmaceutical interests are not the same as patients' interest. Drug companies know physicians in general do not have the time to critically

review medical literature; they rely on summaries. Also, they know that few physicians are skilled in statistics or the necessity of good study design. A good example of deception in drug testing is the well-written book by Peter R. Breggin, MD, *Toxic Psychiatry*, concerning the promotion of drugs used in psychiatry. The lessons learned in that book apply also to all fields of medical research.

4. Individual differences among patients are unpredictable and more common than generally realized. Furthermore, many of the pre-approval appraisals were performed on healthy young adults whereas, in practice, the patient may be a malnourished 85 year-old with a bad liver.

5. The patient may have several doctors, each prescribing drugs without knowledge of or consultations concerning the polypharmacy risk being created. Or, the patient is also taking over-the-counter medications without the doctor's knowledge. The possible drug interactions become unmanageably complex.

6. The patient has been led to believe that the doctor always knows best. But the doctor is also human and, as such, prone to error.

7. The doctor has been trained in a mind-set derived from the "war" against bacterial infections in which success (such as it was) was achieved by a process of diagnosing diseases by their signs and symptoms in order to identify the infecting organism so the proper antibiotic may be employed to kill it. But, today's diseases are of a different sort as we have seen; the "magic bullet" theory doesn't apply. Today's treatments must consider the broad matrix of interrelating factors that affect immune competence, nutritional adequacy, individual genetic and environmental differences, toxins, and viruses for

which no antibiotics yet exist. Doctors must learn to think in terms of intra-cellular metabolic functions rather than superficial manifestations; they must strive to augment natural defenses rather than merely "treat" symptoms; they must educate their patients in matters of nutrition and care of his body rather than wait for disease to become overt. You must understand that doctors are ill prepared by their training to do this.

8. The doctor's required continuing medical education (CME) is often at the hands of the pharmaceutical industry whose business it is to sell their products. Unless constantly mindful, doctors will succumb to the propaganda and believe themselves educated. Not only have they now become part of the problem but the time taken by these pharmaceutical-provided medical seminars reduces the likelihood that they will ever, on their own, get around to learning about the solution such as, for instance, reading *The Kellogg Report: The Impact of Nutrition, Environment & Lifestyle on the Health of Americans*, a 735 page opus from the Institute of Health Policy and Practice.

9. There is the prevalent notion that health is a free ride requiring no effort on our part for it to be achieved. If it ain't broke, don't fix it. As long as you can make it through the day, you're all right. This is nonsense, of course. We do know better but we don't like to think about it. We take care of our cars; why don't we learn how to take care of our bodies? Instead, we wait until something does break down and then expect the doctor to fix it with magic. This is the perfect setting for iatrogenic disease.

10. Iatrogenic medicine also involves governmental medical bureaucracies, such as the Food and Drug Agency, the National Institutes of Health, or the Public Health Service. The nature of bureaucracies is such that being a

"team member" is more highly rewarded than being a dissident. Criticizing the policies of one's superior does not usually strengthen one's career. Thus, an established health policy, whether erroneous or not, tends strongly to become a fixed policy, almost immune to the normal changes and new understandings that regularly occur in general medical practice.

One such example is fluoridation which originated over 50 years ago with the observation that mottled dental enamel was caused by fluoride in drinking water and an apparent (but inadequately tested) correlation of water fluoride with fewer dental cavities in children. Despite protests from many physicians and toxicologists, the addition of fluoride compounds to public water became a fixed policy of the Public Health Service (PHS). Flawed early studies appeared to support this policy. More recent and far better studies have now shown that (1) the decline in children's dental caries is less a function of water fluoridation than of better diet, better dental hygiene, or an acquired immune response to cariogenic plaque bacteria (*Strep mutans*); (2) the toxicity of fluoride is much greater than previously thought, correlated with increased cancer, particularly osteosarcoma [in young males], colon cancer, heart arrhythmia deaths, gastritis, and osteoporotic hip fracture; and (3) the typical total daily intake of fluoride (due to fluoridated water-processing of food and to high fluoride toothpaste) now exceeds known toxic levels in US communities regardless of fluoridation status.

Previously, "optimal" fluoridation (i.e., presumed to be safe) was defined as that intake that caused < 10% of the children to have mottled teeth. The PHS now admits that dental fluorosis is found in 10% of children in *unfluoridated* communities and in 34% of children in *fluoridated* communities. Rather than reducing water fluoride concentrations, the PHS calls for more money for research in decreasing fluoride exposure from other sources such as food-borne and toothpaste fluoride. In this regard, it should be recalled that, for reasons of toxicity and lack of efficacy, Japan, India and all western European countries (except Spain which is still battling over it) have decided against the practice; and Australia now advocates decreasing their fluoride concentration to one-half that of ours. Yet, despite all the evidence against it, our PHS continues to advocate the same fluoridation level as it did in 1943 when food-borne fluoride and fluoridated toothpaste did not exist.

Thus, iatrogenic disease takes many forms. As patients, we must be ever vigilant and not be timid in challenging our health "authorities" to keep up with medical knowledge and to follow the rule of "primum non nocere." It's *our* health, after all.

A FEW EXAMPLES OF IATROGENIC PROBLEMS

1. Between 4-10% of all hospital admissions are due to adverse drug reactions.

2. Over 20% of hospital admissions are due to mismanagement of drugs, either by the patient or the doctor.

3. One study suggests that over-prescription of hypertension drugs may cause 25,000 heart attacks each year. Estimated cost is over $1 *billion*.

4. Side effects of about 70 million prescriptions annually for non-steroidal anti-inflammatory drugs (NSAIDs) include 200-300,000 cases of gastro-intestinal tract bleeding each year, leading to 10-20,000 deaths.

5. Unopposed estrogen is the only known cause of endometrial cancer and probably increases the risk of breast cancer, yet it is widely prescribed to postmenopausal women for hot flashes and retarding osteoporosis. When accompanied by synthetic progestins (to decrease the endometrial cancer risk), these impose a different set of potential adverse side effects.

6. Broad-spectrum antibiotic use predisposes one to secondary yeast infections, loss of "friendly" colon flora (e.g., the ones producing vitamin K for us), and diarrhea. In addition, the more antibiotics used, the more likely is

the development of antibiotic-resistant disease organisms.

7. Certain diuretics (e.g., furosemide [Lasix]) cause urinary loss of calcium and other minerals, leading to increased risk of osteoporosis.

8. We should not forget the DES (diethylstilbestrol) babies that grew up to develop vaginal cancer, the X-radiated thyroid patients that later developed thyroid cancer, the swine flu immunizations that caused Guillian-Barre paralysis, or the thalidomide babies. Quite a long list could be compiled.

The practice of medicine is an incomplete science and there is a long way to go. We have strayed too far down the path of drug manipulation of symptoms; we need to return to the path of prevention. Present paradigms are failing us but an aroused and knowledgeable public can re-direct our efforts along the path of optimal health.

CONCLUSION

Optimal health is not achieved by neglecting the fundamental facts of nature. Our bodies are wondrous, to be sure, but will achieve optimal results only when cared for in optimal fashion. To do this, one does not have to be a biochemist or nutrition scientist; one only has to learn and follow certain basic precepts, which, in ages past, were part of a shared culture and known to all. In our modern technological society, our rate of change has outstripped our cultural knowledge heritage. We must, then, re-learn the lessons of nature..... the wholesome diet, the body's need for exercise, and the limits of stress. To our advantage, the body's signals can be our guide; dysfunction and disease are potent indicators of straying off course. The goal and purpose of this text is to help chart the path to the attainment of our optimal health.

ANSWERS TO SELF QUIZ QUESTIONS

<u>Chapter 9.</u>   1. false, 2. false, 3. HDL, 4. false, 5. sugar and animal fat, among others, 6. true, 7. (c), 8. true, 9. false, 10. true.

<u>Chapter 10.</u>   1. (b) diet, 1. false, 3. potassium, sodium, 4. false, 5. true, 6. true, 7. true, 8. true, 9. false, 10. true.

<u>Chapter 11.</u>   1. false, 2. 5-6 oz protein/day, 3. 30%, 4. 5%, 5. true, 6. false, 7. true, 8. true, 9. true, 10. false.

<u>Chapter 12.</u>   1. true, 2. calcium, 3. osteoblast, 4. progesterone, 5. testosterone, 6. estrogen, 7. true, 8. true, 9. false, 10. true.

<u>Chapter 13.</u>   1. false, 2. false, 3. true, 4. false, 5. (b), 6. (e), 7. Vitamins A, C, and E, and selenium, 8. true, 9. false, 10. true.

<u>Chapter 14.</u>   1. ptyalin, or salivary amylase, 2. true, 3. false, 4. false, 5. truc, 6. cmulsify, 7. true, 8. the gall bladder, 9. false, 10. false.

<u>Chapter 15.</u>   1. true, 2. true, 3. false, 4. true, 5. 76 %, 6. false, 7. false, 8. true, 9. false, 10. false.

GLOSSARY

adrenalin . . . . "fight or flight" hormone secreted by the medulla of the adrenal gland in response to stress or hypoglycemia, activating the sympathetic nervous system to cause increased blood pressure, accelerated heart rate, bronchial dilation, and pupil dilation; also known as epinephrine.

aerobic . . . . lives (or functions) only in the presence of molecular oxygen.

agonist . . . . muscle or biochemical function opposed in action by another muscle or biochemical function called the antagonist.

amino acid . . . . an organic acid containing an amino ($-NH_2$) group; just 22 amino acids make up all the body's proteins.

amygdala . . . . a specific neural nucleus in the limbic brain named for its almond shape; it is the center of our rage response.

amyloid . . . . abnormal complex glycoprotein material found micro-scopically in certain disease states.

anaerobic . . . . can live (or function) without oxygen being present.

analgesic . . . . relieves or not sensitive to pain.

antagonist . . . . that which opposes an agonist (see above).

antibiotic . . . . 1. life destroyer. 2. usually, a chemical substance produced by fungi (or synthetically made) to inhibit or destroy bacteria, used in treatment of infectious dis-eases.

antioxidant . . . . a chemical (e.g. vitamin or mineral) or compound that inhibits oxidation reactions by free radicals.

arteriosclerosis . . . . . . hardening of the arteries.

atherogenic . . . . a process or substance that induces atherosclerosis.

atherosclerosis ...... deposits of cholesterol, lipoid material, and cellular debris in the intima (inner lining) of large and medium-sized arteries.

autoimmune .... the production by an organism of reactivity to its own tissues; an abnormal immune response directed against oneself.

autonomic .... self-controlling; (med) refers to sympathetic and parasympathetic nervous systems.

bacillus .... a rod-shaped bacterium.

bacteria .... unicellular organism of the plant kingdom.

carcinogen .... any cancer-producing substance.

carotid .... pertaining to the principal artery of the neck (carrying blood to the brain).

catabolism .... a process in which complex substances are converted to simpler compounds; considered as destructive metabolism.

catalyst .... any substance that induces a change in velocity or direction of a chemical process without becoming part of the final product.

chlamydia .... a subgroup of Rickettsial microorganisms that can cause eye infections and/or inflammatory pelvic infections.

chromosomes .... paired molecules composed of DNA in the form of a double helix found within a cell's nucleus, segments of which compose the genomes (the individual genetic units). 46 in humans.

chylomicron .... particle of emulsified fat, one micron in diameter, found in blood during digestion of fat.

claudication .... pain or discomfort in a limb occurring after use of the limb and relieved by rest, found in occlusive arterial disease

coccus .... a round or spherical bacterium, usually slightly < 1 μ (micron) in diameter.

collagen .... the main protein of connective tissue, i.e., skin, tendon, bone and cartilage, reduces to gelatin by boiling.

colon .... the large intestine (extends from the cecum to the rectum).

corpus callosum ..... the large transverse bundle of nerves connecting the right and left cerebral hemispheres.

cytoplasm .... the watery protoplasm within a cell.

DES .... diethylstilbestrol, an estrogen used to fatten steers.

differentiation .... the process of developing specialized form or function.

disaccharide .... a compound sugar, composed of two simple sugars (mono- saccharides).

diuretic .... any agent that promotes the secretion of urine.

DNA .... deoxyribonucleic acid, of which chromosomes are made.

eclampsia .... an uncommon condition of late pregnancy, cause unclear, with headache, edema, hypertension, oliguria and proteinuria complicated by seizures and coma.

electrolyte .... minerals or compounds which, when dissolved in water, can conduct electricity.

embryogenesis ...... the embryo (early) stage of the development of a new individual from a fertilized ovum.

endocrine .... pertaining to glands that secrete a substance that has a specific effect on another organ or part e.g., thyroid, ovary.

endometrium .... the inner mucous coat of the uterus.

endorphin .... polypeptide hormone of the central nervous system.

enzyme .... an organic (usually a macro-polypeptide) catalyst.

eosinophile .. .. a leukocyte with red-staining granules in its cytoplasm (the granules contain a lytic substance to dissolve agents interpreted as foreign to the body).

epigenetic .... referring to the area surrounding the genes but not the genes themselves.

epinephrine .... same as adrenalin (Greek-derived name instead of Latin-derived).

erythropoieses .... the production of erythrocytes, i.e., red blood cells.

estrogen . . . . class name of the ovarian hormones that initiate the body's preparation for possible fertilization and pregnancy.

fatty acid . . . . major constituent of fat.

fornix . . . . arch-like; an arched nerve fiber tract directly under the corpus callosum.

free radical . . . . any compound with unbalanced electrons, capable of causing destabilizing oxidation reactions.

gene . . . . the biologic unit of heredity, a segment of DNA, now more often called genome.

genetic . . . . pertaining to reproduction or birth or to heredity.

gram . . . . basic unit of mass (weight) of the metric system; 28.35 grams are equivalent to one ounce (avoirdupois). If one were to cut up a letter that could be mailed for one first class stamp into 28 pieces, each of the pieces would weigh one gram.

hemochromatosis. . . . an inherited (genetic) condition of iron regulation in which dietary iron absorption is greater than body need.

hemolytic . . . . causes hemoglobin to separate from red blood cells.

heterogeneous . . . . consisting of dissimilar elements; not homogeneous.

hippocampus . . . . curved (like a seahorse) nerve structure of the limbic brain, vital to learning and memory.

homeostasis . . . . maintaining a normal, stable internal environment.

hydrogenation . . . . the process of combining with hydrogen.

hydroxyl . . . . the univalent radical (-OH) which, in combination with hydrogen (H), forms water and, in combination with other radicals, forms hydroxides.

hypertension . . . . high blood pressure.

hypoglycemia . . . . low blood sugar level.

hypotension . . . . low blood pressure.

hypothalamus . . . . neural nuclei in the limbic brain just above the pituitary, a major site for physiologic homeostasis.

hysterectomy . . . . surgical removal of the uterus.

iatrogenic . . . . resulting from the actions of physicians.

ischemic . . . . deficient in blood.

Kcal . . . . kilo(thousand)calories, a standard unit of heat, commonly referred to as simply a calorie in the study of metabolism.

lactobacillus acidophilus . . .bacteria that ferment lactose (in milk) to lactic acid and are not destroyed by stomach acid.

legume . . . . vegetables which bear seeds in pods, e.g., peas, beans.

leukocyte . . . . white blood cell.

leukopenia . . . . deficiency in white blood cells (leukocytes).

libido . . . . sexual desire.

limbic brain . . . . the portion of the brain immediately below the corpus callosum and atop the pons; it is the first to receive the ascending spinal cord afferent nerves and is the cerebral center for emotions and homeostasis .

lipoprotein . . . . lipid combined with protein for serum solubility.

mammillary bodies. . . small rounded protrusions of brain cells at the floor of the anterior portion of the limbic brain, possibly integrating sense of smell with sex drive .

menopause . . . . cessation of menstrual cycles.

metabolism . . . . the sum of all biochemical processes by which organisms live, the transformation by which energy is made available for the uses of the organism.

metastasis . . . . the transfer of disease from one organ to another not directly connected with it (as in pathogenic microorganisms or malignant cells).

microgram . . . . one-millionth (10^{-6}) of a gram, or one-thousandth (10^{-3}) of a milligram.

micron . . . . unit of linear measure, one-thousandth (10^{-3}) of a millimeter.

milligram . . . . one-thousandth (10^{-3}) of a gram.

millimeter . . . . one-thousandth (10^{-3}) of a meter; 25.4 to the inch.

mitochondria . . . . small organelles within the cytoplasm that convert glucose bonds into energy; contains its own DNA, different from the nuclear DNA.

mnemonic . . . . memory aid, usually by alphabetic or word cues.

molecule . . . . a combination of two or more atoms which form a specific chemical substance.

myocardium . . . . the heart muscle.

myopathy . . . . any disease of a muscle.

nanogram . . . . one-billionth (10^{-9}) of a gram, a millionth (10^{-6}) of a milligram.

nephro- . . . . pertaining to the kidney.

neurolemma . . . . the myelin layers insulating a nerve fiber.

neuropathy . . . . any disease of nerves.

noradrenalin . . . . modified adrenalin molecule enabling it to pass the blood/brain barrier; also called norepinephrine.

oliguria . . . . production of a diminished amount of urine relative to fluid intake.

omnivore . . . . one whose diet contains both vegetables and meat.

oophorectomy . . . . surgical removal of an ovary.

organelle . . . . small intracellular cytoplasmic structure including mitochondria, the Golgi complexes, ribosomes, and centrioles.

orthostatic . . . . pertaining to change of position, e.g., standing erect.

osteoblast . . . . bone cell that makes new bone.

osteoclast . . . . bone cell that resorbs previously made (old) bone.

osteosarcoma . . . . bone sarcoma (cancer).

paradigm . . . . 1. a list of all inflectional forms of a word taken as illustrative examples of the conjugation or declension to which it belongs, or 2. the various applications of a central concept.

peptide . . . . compounds of low molecular weight, containing two or more amino acids: enzymes are macro-polypeptides.

periarticular . . . . situated around a joint.

petechia . . . . small, pinpoint, round red spot caused by intradermal or subcutaneous hemorrhage.

petrochemical . . . . chemicals derived from petroleum products.

photon . . . . a particle (quantum) of electromagnetic radiation, e.g., of light or X-ray.

plaque . . . . 1. a patch or slightly raised flat area; 2. the visible accumulations of lipoid material within arteries .

polyunsaturated fatty acid . . . a fatty acid with more than one double bond in its carbon chain.

preeclampsia . . . . an uncommon condition of late pregnancy with head- ache, edema, hypertension, oliguria and proteinuria; cause unclear.

progesterone . . . . the ovarian hormone made by the corpus luteum (after ovulation) to sustain luteal-phase endometrium and support a potential fertilized ovum and embryogenesis.

progestin . . . . a synthetic compound with progesterone-like action on the luteal-phase endometrium.

prostaglandin . . . . class of hormone composed of essential fatty acids with effects on smooth muscle contraction and cellular inflammation responses (originally found in semen).

prostate . . . . the male gland surrounding the neck of the bladder and urethra; prepares fluid mixed with sperm for ejacula- tion.

protozoa . . . . unicellular organisms of the animal kingdom.

pylorus . . . . distal neck of the stomach through which gastric contents pass into the duodenum.

radical . . . . in chemistry, a group of atoms which enters into and goes out of chemical combinations without change, and which forms one of the fundamental constituents of a molecule (e.g., -OH).

RNA . . . . ribonucleic acid which transfers information from DNA to protein-forming systems within a cell; composed of nucleic acids adenine, guanine, cytosine, and uracil plus ribose and phosphoric acid (as does DNA).

saccharide . . . . carbohydrate molecule of which sugar is composed.

saturated fatty acid . . . fatty acid with full complement of hydrogen, i.e., no double bond in the carbon chain of the fatty acid.

scurvy . . . . disease of connective tissue deterioration due to vitamin C deficiency.

sterol . . . . fat soluble monohydroxy alcohol compound composed of hydrocarbon rings, e.g., cholesterol .

streptococcus . . . . genus of cocci microorganisms which include a number of animal pathogens.

synergy . . . . coordinated or cooperative action of two or more structures or active compounds such that their combined effect is greater than the algebraic sum of their individual actions.

synthesis . . . . "putting together," the building of a chemical compound by the union of its elements.

teleologic . . . . pertaining to design or purpose of natural processes or occurrences.

thalamus . . . . a major limbic brain neural nucleus, the main relay center for sensory impulses to the cerebral cortex.

triglyceride. . . . . a fat composed of glycerin (3-carbon chain) and 3 fatty acids.

trophic . . . . of or pertaining to nutrition.

tuber. . . . . *anatomy*, swelling or protuberance; *botany*, a swollen, usually underground stem, such as a potato, bearing buds from which new shoots arise.

unsaturated fatty acid fatty acid with at least one double bond in the carbon chain.

vasoactive . . . . having an action on veins or arteries, e.g., constriction or dilatation.

vasodilator. . . . . an agent, as a nerve or drug, that dilates arteries.

(202)

PARTIAL BIBLIOGRAPHY

Bailey, C. (1977) *Fit or Fat?* Houghton Mifflin Company, Boston.

Barnard, Neal D. (1992) *The Power of Your Plate*, available from Physicians Committee for Responsible Medicine, P.O. Box 6322, Washington DC.

Beasley, J. D. and Swift, J. J. (1989) *The Kellogg Report: the impact of nutrition, environment and lifestyle on the health of Americans.* The Institute of Health Policy and Practice, The Bard College Center.

Bland, J. edit. (1983) *Medical Applications of Clinical Nutrition.* Keats Pub. New Canaan, Conn.

Breggin, P. R. (1991) *Toxic Psychiatry.* St. Martin's Press, New York.

Brunswick, J. P., Love, D., Weinberg, A. (1977) *How To Live 365 Days A Year The Salt-free Way.* Bantam Books, NYC, NY.

Carlson, R. and Shield, B. eds. *Healers on Healing* (1989), published by Jeremy P. Tarcher, Inc. (St. Martin's Press, distributor)

Cameron, E., and Pauling, L. (1979) *Cancer And Vitamin C.* The Linus Pauling Institute of Science and Medicine, Menlo Park, CA.

Cheraskin, E. and Ringsdorf, W. M. (1973) *Predictive Medicine: A Study in Strategy.* Pacific Press Pub. Co., Mountain View, CA.

Cheraskin, E. and Ringsdorf, W. M. (1984) *The Vitamin C Connection.* Bantam Books, NYC, NY.

Colborn, T., Dumanoski, D., and Myers, J. P. *Our Stolen Future.* Penguin, NY, NY.

Conner, K. H. (1968) *Aerobics.* Bantam Books, NYC, NY.

Dickey, L. D. edit. (1976) *Clinical Ecology.* Charles C. Thomas, Springfield, IL.

Erasmus, U. (1994) *Fats That Heal, Fats That Kill.* alive books, Vancouver, British Columbia.

Ferguson, M. (1973) *The Brain Revolution.* Bantam Books, NYC, NY.

Hoffer, A. and Walker, M. (1978) *Orthomolecular Nutrition.* Keats Pub.,New Canaan, Conn.

Hunter, B. T. (1975) *Food Additives and Federal Policy: The Mirage of Safety.* Charles Scribner's Sons, NYC, NY.

Kirschmann, J. D. and Dunne, L. J. (1984) *Nutrition Almanac,* 2nd Edition. McGraw-Hill Book Co., New York and San Francisco.

Lappe, F. M. (1982) *Diet for a Small Planet,* Revised. Ballantine Books, NY.

Lee, J.R. (1993) *Natural Progesterone: the Multiple Roles of a Remarkable Hormone.* BLL Publishing, Box 2068, Sebastopol, CA 95473

Lee, J. R. and Hopkins, V. (1996) *What Your Doctor May Not Tell You About Menopause.* Warner Books, New York.

Lee J. R., Hanley, J., and Hopkins, V. (1999) *What Your Doctor May Not Tell You About Premenopause.* Warner Books, New York.

Mandell, M. and Scanlon, L. W. (1979) *5-Day Allergy Relief System.* Pocket Books, NYC.

McDougall, J. M. (1985) *McDougall's Medicine: A Challenging Second Opinion.* New Win Publishing, Inc.

McDougall, J. M. (1990) *The McDougall Program.* A Plum Book (Penguin).

National Academy of Sciences (1971) *FLUORIDES,* Washington D.C

Ornish, D. (1982) *Stress, Diet, & Your Heart.* Signet Books, New York.

Pauling, L. (1986) *How to Live Longer and Feel Better.* Avon Books, NY, NY.

Pfeiffer, C. C. and Brain Bio Center. (1975) *Mental and Elemental Nutrients.* Keats Pub., New Canaan, Conn.

Pfeiffer, C. C. (1978) *Zinc and Other Micro-nutrients.* Keats Pub., New Canaan, Conn.

Quillin, P. (1987) Healing Nutrients. Contemporary Books, Chicago, New York.

Roberts, H. J. (audiocassette) *Is Aspartame (NutraSweet®) Safe?* Sunshine Sentinal Press, Inc., P.O. Box 8697-S, West Palm Beach, FL 33407.

Robbins, J. (1987) *Diet For A New America.* Stillpoint Pub., Walpole, NH.

Robin, E. D. (1984) *Matters of Life & Death: Risks vs. Benefits of Medical Care.* The Portable Stanford, Stanford, CA.

Selye, H. (1956) *The Stress of Life.* McGraw-Hill Book Co., New York, Toronto, London.

Selye, H. (1974) *Stress Without Distress.* J. P. Lippincott Co., NYC, NY.

Sheinkin, D., Schachter, M., Hutton, R. (1979) *Food, Mind and Mood.* Warner Books, NYC, NY.

Steingraber, S. (1998) *Living Downstream.* Vintage Books, a division of Random House, Inc., New York.

Stone, I. (1972) *The Healing Factor: "Vitamin C" Against Disease.* Grosset & Dunlop, NY.

Thomas, L. (1974) *The Lives of a Cell.* Viking Press, New York.

Thomas, L. (1979) *The Medusa and the Snail.* Viking Press, New York.

Thomas, L. (1984) *The Youngest Science.* Bantam Books, New York.

Thomas, J. H., Gillham, B. (1989) *Wills' Biochemical Basis of Medicine*, second edition, Wright publishing, London.

Waldbott, G. L., Burgstahler A.W., McKinney H.L. (1978) *Fluoridation: The Great Dilemma.* Coronado Press, Inc., Lawrence, Kansas.

Weil, A. (1990) *Natural Health, Natural Medicine.* Houghton Mifflin Co., Boston.

Williams, R. J. and Kalita, D.K. (1977) *A Physician's Handbook on Orthomolecular Medicine.* Pergamon Press, New York and Toronto.

Williams, R. J. (1973) *Nutrition Against Disease*. Bantam Books, NYC, NY.

Williams, R. J. (1977) *The Wonderful World Within You*. Bantam Books, NYC, NY.

Yiamouyiannis, J. (1983) *Fluoride: The Aging Factor*. Health Action Press, Delaware, Ohio.

INDEX